Taking Care of Mama

by

Ellen Abel

Bloomington, IN  Milton Keynes, UK

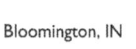

AuthorHouse™
1663 Liberty Drive, Suite 200
Bloomington, IN 47403
www.authorhouse.com
Phone: 1-800-839-8640

AuthorHouse™ UK Ltd.
500 Avebury Boulevard
Central Milton Keynes, MK9 2BE
www.authorhouse.co.uk
Phone: 08001974150

This book is a work of non-fiction. Unless otherwise noted, the author and the publisher make no explicit guarantees as to the accuracy of the information contained in this book and in some cases, names of people and places have been altered to protect their privacy.

First published by AuthorHouse 11/14/2006

ISBN: 978-1-4259-6202-9 (sc)

Library of Congress Control Number: 2006907902
Printed in the United States of America
Bloomington, Indiana

This book is printed on acid-free paper.

My worst nightmare was to have my mother die…

Amanda Williams had a passion for family love and togetherness, and for helping anyone in need. Her strong character impacted the lives of all she came in contact with.

She also had Alzheimer's Disease.

This is her story.

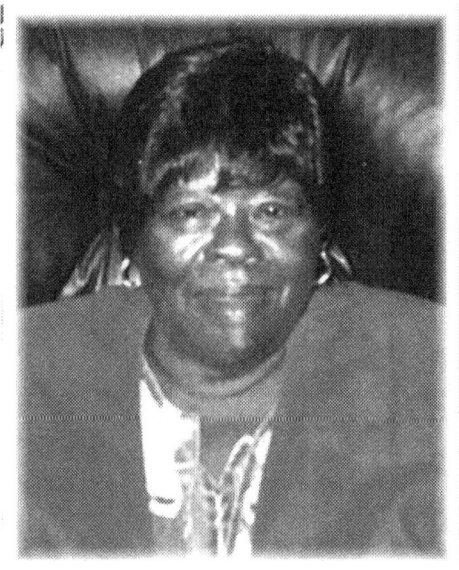

DEDICATION

I WOULD LIKE TO DEDICATE THIS BOOK TO MY MOTHER, AMANDA WILLIAMS, WHO DIED ON OCTOBER 15, 2004. MAMA LEFT A LEGACY OF FAMILY, LOVE, AND TOGETHERNESS, AND OF HELPING ANYONE THAT NEEDED HER HER CHARACTER .HAD AN IMPACT ON EVERYONE WHO CAME IN CONTACT WITH HER. SHE TRIED TO ENCOURAGE EVERYONE WHO KNEW HER TO LOVE EACH OTHER.

MAMA WILL BE MISSED BUT NEVER FORGOTTEN. SHE WILL ALWAYS BE IN THE HEARTS OF THOSE WHO KNEW AND LOVED HER.

I ALSO DEDICATE THIS BOOK TO THE FRIENDS AND, FAMILIES — AND ESPECIALLY THE CHILDREN OF — ALZHEIMER'S VICTIMS COPING WITH THE EMOTIONAL STRESS OF MANAGING CARE FOR THE ALZHEIMER'S SUFFERER.

ACKNOWLEDGMENT

I would like to express my thanks and gratitude to my daughter, Chekena Carter, who always supports me and takes great interest in all my endeavors.

I would like to thank VITAS for being there for me and my family when we needed them most, VITAS is an organization that works with hospice patients; they were a tremendous help in our time of need.

I am grateful to my sisters, Clara Foster and Karen Howard, for reminding me to take time for myself when I got so stressed from dealing with the emotional difficulties Mama was enduring. They made sure that I spent some time out of the house and away from the situation —sometimes dinner, sometimes a movie, and sometimes just a sisters gathering gave the whole ordeal balance.

I thank Kim Seaton and Rhonda Burchman for hiring me at Sun View Care Center, and for allowing me to get the firsthand experience I needed by working there, to be better equipped to take care of Mama, and for being so very understanding when I needed to take time off from work to see about my mother in Florida.

I also thank Donna Gilroy for working with me and helping me adapt to the Alzheimer's residents on Valencia Villa.

Thank you, Pastor Ernest Cobbs, for uplifting our family during our time of grief, and for lifting our spirits, and for reminding us of the good times that we had with Mama. Thank you, Pastor Cobbs, for being there for our family as you have been in the past when we needed your kind and compassionate words to keep us strong

Thank you, David Shenk (the author of *The Forgetting*), for writing this national bestseller. It helped me understand

Mama's new personality or mood swings, and was a guide for me when she was going through her stages of dementia.

Thank you, Meg Basset for the cover design ideas you so brilliantly put together on a moments notice, Meg is a Painter a Nurse , and a good friend .

INTRODUCTION

My worst nightmare was to have my mother die, leaving me in this world without her.

Having to wake up each day knowing that Mama had died would have killed me or I would have lost my mind. (Even as an adult, I had these fears.)

But Mama did die, and as you can see, it didn't kill me. And yes, Mama did leave me, and I didn't lose my mind. GOD does not let us endure any more than we can handle.

Before Mama died, she developed Alzheimer's disease. It took away her character, her personality and her spirit. That was almost as devastating as Mama dying. Those were the parts of Mama I loved the most.

Although Alzheimer's disease was known about for many years, knowledge about its causes, treatment, and the care of the people with the disease was slow in developing. Only recently, research on behavioral, social, and environmental aspects of the disease have caused attitudes to begin to change.

Mentally, Mama had slipped away from me, and I was left with a deteriorating stranger who was supposed to be Mama, but she was all I had to hang on to. I was going through the worst storm of my life, it seemed, and I prayed that GOD would change my circumstances, and change the situation, but he was silent. I couldn't even feel his presence; I felt like I had to go it alone.

I later learned that in times such as these, you have to trust GOD and have confidence in him. He will see you through all of your troubles. No matter how low your valleys seem to be, GOD knows how it's going to turn out, because he's already seen your tomorrow.

When I finally realized that I had to accept the things that I couldn't change, Mama was getting weaker but I was getting stronger.

As I prepared myself to return to Florida, I bought a journal, because I knew that I wouldn't be able to talk to Daddy about Mama's situation; he was in denial regarding Mama's mental state. Daddy saw a completely different picture than the one I was looking at. He assumed that with a little TLC from me Mama would be all right.

After Mama died, and it didn't kill me and I didn't lose my mind, I decided to write this book from my journal. But before I talk about taking care of Mama, I'd like to reflect on Mama's life before she got sick.

TAKING CARE OF MAMA
CHAPTER ONE

"Amanda Hannah Williams" was Mama's maiden and married name. But by family, friends, and people who knew and loved her. She was called by many names: Mom, Mama, Manda, Ms. Manda, Aunt Snook, Nanny Snook, or Nana Snook. Mama answered to each of these names and she represented someone special to each person who called her a different name.

In a family as big as ours, that can be one heck of a job, and when you add in the people who loved and depended on her, Mama spread herself pretty thin.

Mama was born into a very large family. She was the eleventh child of sixteen brothers and sisters. She was born in Tallahassee, Florida, where she was also married to my father, Robert Williams, at a very young age. Daddy was born in Georgia, but his family moved to Tallahassee. After Mom and Dad were married, Daddy enlisted in the military. When he returned to Tallahassee, he and Mom moved to Miami, Florida, where they were blessed with five daughters: my sisters Annette, Bobbie, Clara, and Karen, and myself, Ellen. I was the third daughter. Mama was happily married to Dad for sixty-five years, and they still loved each other.

Mama has always been a shining star in my eyes, ever since I can remember her.

When Mama was a young woman, she was very pretty. She had high cheekbones, with smooth brown skin, beautiful eyes, and a healthy head of hair. Mama stood about 5 feet 5, 130 pounds, and her eyes lit up every time she flashed her beautiful smile.

Mama was a fun-loving person. She loved being around her children, her family, and her friends. She loved music, dancing, and having fun. Mama was active in our community. I believe her calling was to be a social worker, or a public relations person. Although Mama didn't finish high school to prepare and enhance what was already inside of her, she didn't let that stop her; she still used the gifts that GOD blessed her with.

Mama was always willing to take some of the neighbors to the store, or if some of them had lost their jobs, she'd make sure that their children would eat at least one hot meal a day (and two if she had enough).

I remember the family who lived across the street from us. They were a family of ten — the parents and eight children. Their father was a blues singer and he played the piano in a band, but he was out of work most of the time. The younger kid, Ronnie, would always come to our house around dinnertime. Ronnie would ask Mama if she would give him a sandwich or something because he was hungry. Mama would make Ronnie a big peanut butter and jelly sandwich. He'd would smile and rub his hands on his too-tight short pants, take the sandwich from Mama, and run out of the front door.

Before we could finish dinner, three more little curly-headed boys (Ronnie's brothers) would stand in front of our screen door and press their dirty little faces into the screen as they called out to Mama.

"Ms. Manda! Ms. Manda! Can we have a samitch, too?"

When Mama opened the front door, she'd look down at their hungry little eyes and serious faces and smile. They would look up at Mama, and then into the kitchen, where we all sat around the table eating dinner. Their mother seemed to always dress them all alike, with tight short pants, and never a shirt or shoes unless it was cold (which was very seldom).

Mama would open the cabinet, take the peanut butter and jelly down again, make three sandwiches, and give them to the boys. Then Mama would pull out a brown paper bag and put the rest of the bread and the peanut butter and jelly into it, and she'd walk the boys to the door and call their sister from our front porch.

"Barbra Jean!" Mama would call out.

"Yes, ma'am, I'm coming." Barbara would answer. As soon as she heard her name called, she knew that Mama was sending something for the rest of them to eat. (The way she'd come running out of the house, and across the street, you'd think Jesus had called her.) When Mama stood on the porch with the brown bag swinging in her hand, the other little ones would tear out behind Barbara and they would all follow her

across the street and stop on our porch shouting, "Ms. Manda! I want some, too!"

"Now, Barbara Jean, you fix the rest of y'all a sandwich," Mama demanded. Sometimes I could see the older kids watching from their front room window, waiting for Barbara Jean to bring the brown paper bag into the house to see if she had enough for them to eat, too.

Despite the hardships our family had, Mama was always a pillar of strength to lean on for everybody else. Mama even opened up our house to abused wives. The lady who lived next door, Ms. Emma, had a bad-tempered husband who'd beat her up all of the time and she'd always run to our house for refuge. Mama would help Ms. Emma by bandaging her bruised arms and legs. Mama kept Ms. Emma safe until her husband cooled off.

Sometimes, Mama would even have to fix up a makeshift bed on the floor in the living room for Ms. Emma. She'd sleep there overnight when her husband had been drinking a lot. I remember the last time Ms. Emma ran to our house. Daddy insisted that she call her family. Later that night, they took Ms. Emma wherever she said she wanted to go. They dropped her off and I never saw her again.

Ms. Emma's husband blamed Mama for ruining their marriage. He never took the blame for any part of their marriage breaking up. Mama told Ms. Emma's husband that he should have been a man instead of hitting on women. Daddy said that he was afraid to face another man, that's why he never came to our house to get his wife.

Mama was a very frank, get-right-to-the-point, kind of person. She didn't do a song and a dance just to tell you what she thought about something. And after she'd told you what she thought about any situation, it was forgotten as far as Mama was concerned.

(MOVING ON)

I thank Mama for some of the fond memories I still have of Christmas, Easter, Thanksgiving, and even the summers we spent together.

Some of my fondest memories are of the nights before Thanksgiving Day; I enjoyed that as much as I enjoyed Thanksgiving Day. Every year, Mama would prepare the Thanksgiving turkey and get some of the side dishes ready the night before Thanksgiving Day (so that all she had to do was put them in the oven on Thanksgiving morning). Our house would have the smell of good spices, poultry seasoning, cinnamon, sweet potato pies, and cakes.

There were five of us girls at the time. Annette was the oldest, but she was already married and had a baby who kept her busy, and Karen was our baby sister, so they just watched. Bobbie, Clara, and I all helped Mama in preparing the meal.

She gave each of us something to do. Someone would chop the veggies while someone mixed the batter for the cornbread (that Mama would use later for cornbread dressing), and I always got to mix the batter for the sweet potato pies.

Daddy's job was to play the music for Mama. He'd play all of the songs Mama liked to hear. Sometimes, Daddy would play a song that Mama really liked, and she would sing and dance all over the kitchen while she continued to cook. Daddy would laugh and tell Mama how good she looked dancing.

Our house was so small that when you walked into the front door, you had a view of our entire house. The only rooms that had doors were the bedrooms and the bathrooms. Daddy could see what we were doing in the kitchen from where he sat in the living room. He played records for Mama to dance to. Daddy would tell the three of us girls that he knew it was going to be a very good Thanksgiving dinner, because we'd done such a good job of chopping and mixing, and helping Mama in the kitchen.

On Thanksgiving Day, it was all about laughing, eating, and having fun, because Mama had prepared a wonderful dinner for us, and made sure everyone was happy. Mama always looked forward to celebrating the holidays. It was one more reason to get the family together, one more reason to prepare a good meal, and one more reason to fill our house with relatives, music, and laughter. It's been hard, but it's a tradition I've tried to keep.

Mama also enjoyed entertaining her friends. Sometimes on the weekends, Mama would entertain her friends with a party. They'd put all of the kids into a room to play. When we got bored, we'd peep out of the door to watch Mama and her friends dance and enjoy themselves. Sometimes, Mama would come into the room and get one of us to go out into the living room to dance with her and sometimes, she'd just tell us to dance for her and her friends, and that was the part of the evening we'd all look forward to.

CHAPTER TWO

FAMILY TIES AND TRADITIONS

As we grew up and got older, Mama made sure we knew how to keep ourselves groomed, and how to clean the house, cook, and take of the younger ones.

Mama made sure that we went to church on Sunday. She taught us to love GOD and keep him first in our lives. Mama would always say that she grew up in a Baptist home, but when she married Daddy, she had to change to his denomination, which was Catholic and that's how we were raised. Even though Mama changed to the Catholic faith, she would still sing her old Baptist hymns around the house when she was cleaning, or when she washed and hung out the clothes on the clothesline. You could hear Mama's voice echoing throughout the neighborhood.

I wished I'd paid more attention to Mama when she tried to teach us who was who in the Bible; she always said that God had a plan for all of us. Maybe if I had listened, I would have made better choices and decisions for myself. During those years, to me, GOD was just some far-off historical person Mama used to keep us in line. I thought I had all the answers, but was I ever wrong. Mama always said we all had to answer to GOD for ourselves, and that it was her job to point us in the right direction.

Mama was always proud of all of her girls no matter what. When our oldest sister Annette got pregnant at a very early age, Mama said even though Annette had broken her heart, she still loved her. When Annette got pregnant, Mama also made sure that she was married before her baby was born. Back in the day they called it a "shotgun wedding." I'm not saying if it was right or not, but as far as Mama was concerned, if you wanted to have a baby, then you needed to have a husband. So Mama made sure that if we got pregnant, we were married by any means necessary.

Mama taught Annette how to be a loving and caring mother. Mama also taught her to be responsible for her own decisions and actions. Even after Annette was married to her husband, she lived in our house — husband, baby, and all.

I was angry all of the time in those days, because there were too many people living in a house that small.

"Why can't they just get their own apartment?" I'd complain.

Mama explained that they couldn't afford a place of their own yet. Before Annette brought her little family into our house, we had our own beds, even if it was in the same room. And of course, Mama and Dad shared a room. After Annette's baby was born, she and her husband moved into the only other bedroom in the house, and the rest of us got kicked out of our bedroom and onto the couch to sleep at night.

We finally moved out of the old neighborhood, and I was glad to leave. Annette and her family continued to live in the little house I hated so much. When we moved, Daddy rented that old house out to Annette and her husband Al for whatever he could afford to pay. Annette cried the day we moved away and into our new house. She wanted to go with us, but Mama said even though she was only sixteen, she'd had a baby and it was time for her to be her own woman.

"I was only fourteen when I got married, and it wasn't 'cause I had a baby; it was time for me to get married," Mama told Annette. "We had a big family and it was time for me to leave."

Everybody cried that day when we had to leave Annette behind; everybody, that is, except Daddy. I didn't think Daddy even knew how to cry.

After we moved and were settled into our new house, Annette had her husband Al drive her across town to our house to visit every Friday. When it was time for them to go home, she would cry. Mama tried to comfort Annette as she helped her pack up to leave. I loved my sister but I was glad to see them go. We had our own beds again, and this, time we had three bedrooms. I was excited about sharing a room with only one sister.

We finally had our own space. We didn't have to bump into each other just to get to the next room. I never wanted things to go back to being the way they were in our old house, not ever again. It was bad enough that we had to endure Daddy's rules I felt that we should at least have our own space when we wanted to pout.

Mama was a hard worker. When she moved to Miami in the 1940s, she started out doing housework, then she became a factory worker as a garment presser. Mama worked on a steam iron machine, and it wore her hip and knee down over a period of time. She began to have problems with her right hip and knee. Because of the kind of machine Mama worked with, she had to stand up all day, using her hip and knee to operate the steam peddle on the machine that she used to pressed each garment with. After many years of pressing in that factory, Mama began to walk with a small limp on her right side. Mama finally had to retire from her job before she really wanted to. She could no longer work in her condition.

CHAPTER THREE

TEENAGE YEARS AND DADDY'S RULES

In the sixties, the three older girls were still living at home. We were in high school. We were trying very hard to develop our own personalities, while at the same time, trying to escape some of Daddy's house rules.

Mama was always there for us, but she had a stubborn streak in her, too. She knew what we were up to most of the time, but sometimes she got it wrong, and we'd get punished for something she thought we'd done. When Mama would realize she was wrong, she'd never apologize, but she'd have a look on her face that said it all; I could tell by the look in her eyes that she knew she'd made a mistake, but she was an adult and adults didn't have to say I'm sorry, and since that's the way things were back then, we just moved on.

Daddy had some pretty strict house rules, and he expected everyone to honor them. When Annette got pregnant, Daddy changed a lot. Every young male in the neighborhood became a suspect as far as Daddy was concerned, but not just because of Annette's pregnancy. Daddy said that they were all after the rest of his daughters. None of the guys on our block would stop or even slow down when they got in front of our house. They said that Daddy was crazy.

Every female in our house was put on lockdown. No one could either come or go unless Daddy said that we could. Daddy was basically a quiet man. He stood about six feet tall, and weighed two hundred ten pounds. He was very light-skinned, had brown hair and close-set dark eyes. Across his forehead, he had frown lines, which made him look like he was mad all of the time. Daddy was the kind of person you didn't want to make angry. He could make life very unpleasant for you.

The older we got, the more it took to take care of us. Daddy worked two jobs, and Mama was on disability. Although Mama was in pain a lot, it never kept her from noticing our personal needs. Mama was always there for us and she knew how we felt about Daddy's rules. Daddy didn't even allow us to get phone calls from boys or even date until we were sixteen. Daddy said that by that time we'd be able to make sound and mature decisions. Daddy always told us that if a young lady stayed out after ten, she was looking for trouble… and if she stayed out after twelve, she'd find it.

I didn't know what kind of trouble Daddy thought we'd run into, but finding him at the front door after twelve would be more trouble than I was willing to face. I never stayed out after twelve.

Mama knew how we felt about Daddy's strict house rules. Daddy had a job during the day, but he also worked at night, so Mama would bend the rules a little when he wasn't there. Mama allowed us to date and have phone calls a little earlier than Daddy's rules permitted us to. Mama often reminded us that Daddy had set such strict rules because he loved us, and he believed that if we followed the rules, they'd keep us out of trouble (or from ending up like our sister Annette).

"It's a mean world out there; you'll find out one day," she'd always tell us.

When we'd come home from school, we could always find Mama in the backyard hanging out a load of clothes on the clothesline each day, and there was always good aromas coming from the oven; most of the time it would be what looked and taste like cake, but Mama said it was a sweet bread. She'd always say to us, "Y'all cut yourself a big ole piece of that sweet bread cause it'll hold you over till your Daddy come home." No one ever ate dinner until Daddy came home.

During my teenage years, I (more than any of my sisters), had a big problem with Daddy's rules, but I managed somehow to keep from fighting with him. I left home right after graduation. I thought that I was grown and wasn't going to put up with Daddy's rules any longer. I ran away and went to Detroit to be with my boyfriend, Jay. He was from Miami, where we met and dated but in my last year of high school. Jay had to go to Detroit to help manage his family's business. When I graduated, I followed him to Detroit.

Although my decision to leave home caused Mama a lot of pain and sickness, Mama was there for me once again. When she found out where I was, she forgave me and wanted to take me back home. Once she learned that I was going to have a baby, and that I didn't want to go back home with her, she said okay. She asked Jay what his intentions were, and she made sure that I was married before she left Detroit. But Mama also made sure that I knew that I could always go back home if I needed to. For a couple of years, my husband and I lived in Detroit (where our oldest daughter was born). We moved back to Miami, Florida, when my husband's coworkers for the General Motors Company went on strike.

While in Miami I had three other children. Unfortunately, my husband and I separated and then divorced. Mama took care of my kids while I went to nursing school (but, I was unable to finish nursing school do to some circumstances beyond my control). With the training that I had, I got a job and was able to support all of us. There were times when I was a young woman, I'd get out of control and do some crazy things but Mama was always able to get me back on track to do what I was suppose to do.

CHAPTER FOUR

JOY, PAIN, SUNSHINE, AND RAIN

By the time the mid-eighties through the nineties rolled around, everyone had either left home or gotten married. We were all involved and tied up in managing our own lives. Mama and dad even celebrated their fiftieth wedding anniversary. When they got remarried, Daddy was finally financially able to give Mama the wedding he'd always wanted for her.

My four sisters and I were Mama's bridesmaids, and each of our oldest daughters were the flower girls.

They were married in St. Mary's Cathedral, and when the priest married them, Mama's eyes sparkled and lit up like a young schoolgirl's.

Although we were all out of the house, and living our own lives, Mama still tried to fix our mistakes when we were having problems. Annette was the oldest. She had five daughters and had divorced their father. Mama was there to get her back on the right track. A few years had passed and Annette got married again. Although she didn't make a very good choice in choosing the second husband, Mama was there to see her through that ordeal.

Bobbie was next in line; she had a beautiful daughter and a wonderful son, whom she and her husband were very proud of. Saudia, Bobbie's daughter, is the mother of three sons. Anon, her son, is a skilled barber. Bobbie didn't give Mama much trouble; she seemed to do the things I always wanted to do, but was never able to achieve.

Clara married her high school sweetheart, William Foster. They became proud parents of their daughter, Kendra.

Unfortunately, they were later divorced. Ten years later, her son Brandon was born. Clara's daughter, Kendra, is the mother of two sons and a daughter Clare. Her son, Brandon, is a student at Clark University. Mama took care of Brandon when he was a baby, and she turned him into a little old man.

Karen, our baby sister had a daughter, Amanda, who was named after Mama. Karen was later married. She and her husband have two wonderful children together and they live in Broward County, Florida.

Mama still kept the family together even though we'd moved out, and were on our own. Everyone loved the way Mama always smoothed out our personal problems and differences. No matter what the problem was, Mama had a way of making us look at ourselves before we blamed the other person. Even when she told us how much of a problem we were to the situation, we knew that she was right. And we did whatever Mama told us to do.

Our ex-husbands and/or boyfriends still came around to visit Mama, even after we had divorced them or our relationships were over. We never had any brothers, so Mama said that they were the sons that she never had, and they loved her for it.

Mama had two total hip operations, but she was still going strong. Even when she realized that she was going to have to use a cane to get around, she saw a brighter side of the situation and found a reason to praise GOD.

In 1979, Annette's third oldest daughter died of an unknown illness and it took a lot out of her. Mama tried to comfort her but it was not enough to replace her lost. In 1984, Annette lost another daughter to AIDS. The news of her daughter having AIDS — and later dying from it — just about killed her. Mama did all she could to comfort Annette again, but her pain was overwhelming; it was too hard for her to accept.

Annette couldn't get over her daughter's death and began having heart problems; she was only forty-seven years old. She had two open-heart surgeries, and a year after the last surgery, she died from complications.

This time, someone needed to be there to comfort Mama. Everyone tried to comfort Mama through her pain, but I guess there is nothing that can fill the void of losing your child to death. Even though we thought Mama had bounced back, she was never quite the same. That sparkle in Mama's eyes had dimmed and it was as though a part of Mama had died with my sister. Although Mama wasn't the same anymore, we still tried to go on with our lives as though nothing had happened; no one talked about it.

Ten years to the exact date of Annette's death, my sister Bobbie was killed in an automobile accident.

An eighteen-wheeler ran her off of the freeway and she went through the windshield and broke her neck. Bobbie was forty-seven years old. Bobbie's death put about ten years on Mama: she looked old and tired. Mama didn't care about too much of anything anymore. The sparkle in Mama's bright eyes had dimmed when Annette died, but after Bobbie was killed, the sparkle was completely gone.

The holidays didn't mean anything to Mama anymore. So we'd invite her and Daddy to our home for the holidays. Everyone saw the change in Mama but no one wanted to talk about it. Even when I tried to address the problem, Daddy would just say to me, "No use talking about something we can't change."

Everyone said that I was making a big deal out of the situation. I was experiencing menopause at the time so I thought maybe I was making too much of it. I thought it was my "mood swings." I had not experienced anything like menopause before, and Bobbie's death caused me to have even more out-of-control emotions. Sometimes I'd cry at the drop of a hat.

17

Bobbie's death affected me almost as much as it did Mama. I thought about everything that had happened: My sisters had died in the order that they were born; Annette was the oldest, and she died first at age forty-seven. She was ten years older than Bobbie, who was born next. Ten years later, she was killed in an accident at age forty-seven. So being the next oldest of the five sisters (and since I was born only one year after Bobbie, I knew that I'd be next in line to die from this curse that I thought had come over our family).

I left my job, my house, friends, and family — all the people who cared about me — so that I could get ready to die. I decided to visit all of my children and grandchildren just in case something had happened to me before I saw them again.

I went to Beaufort, South Carolina to visit Kena, my youngest daughter and her family. Then, I went to Charlotte, North Carolina. I had some serious issues when I got to Charlotte and I was trying to sort them out. My oldest daughter tried to convince me to see someone about my problem.

I didn't have GOD in my life then, so I was drinking, and thinking, and letting the devil fill my mind with all kinds of things. I'd convinced myself that our whole family would be wiped out because of this curse that I'd made up in my head and put on our family — that we were all going to die in the order that we were born. I drank, cried, and imagined all kind of foolishness all day. I even thought about the things I was going to do later in life and places I wanted to go and see; none of these thoughts had entered my mind before, but the more Hennessy I drank, the more things I found to cry about. Finally, the list of things I wanted to do and places I wanted to go was much longer than the things I'd already done. I cried some more because, in my mind, I'd be dead before I had a chance to do anything on the list.

I later realized that if I'd paid attention to what Mama tried to teach me about praying and learning the scriptures, I'd have had a different frame of mind to help me through those times, and I wouldn't have been so depressed. I should have been trying to get direction GOD instead of drinking and drowning in my own sorrow.

(SEPTEMBER 1996)

CHARLOTTE, NORTH CAROLINA

It had rained all morning, and by twelve o'clock, there was still no sun in the sky. When I looked out of my daughter Chris's back door, I could see the gray September sky and the lifeless trees and dead leaves that could lend no hand in cheering me up. As far as I could see in the distance, everything out there was either dead or dying, and that's the way I saw myself. I couldn't stop thinking what was going to happen to me, how was I going to die? Would it be my blood pressure that would take me out or some kind of accident? It was the most depressing day I'd had since I'd been there.

My birthday would be coming around in two weeks. On October 11, I'd be forty-seven years old. "Only forty-seven and it'll be my time to die," I kept thinking. My two older sisters had died at age forty-seven, and I'd be next.

Chris had been watching me and saw how depressed I'd become. She suggested again that I be seen by a doctor, just to talk about my depression. After a long discussion, I agreed to see someone. I'd always taken pride in keeping my hair nice, but two weeks before my birthday, I cut all of the hair off of my head. I was really losing it; my thinking was not rational. I said to myself, "I'm going to die anyway, so what's the use in spending money on my hair? I'm just going to cut it all off and be done with it."

When Chris came home from work that day and looked at my head, it was apparent to her that I needed to see someone sooner than we thought. Chris called a family health clinic and made an appointment for me to see someone about my problem.

The day that I had an appointment, I watched The Oprah Winfrey Show while waiting for my daughter to drive me to the doctor's office. Patti LaBelle was on the Oprah show, and she talked about how her sisters had died one after the other, and how concerned she was. Except for the age thing with my sisters all dying at age forty-seven, Patty seemed to have had the same problem with her sisters all dying one after the other. She said that she prayed and trusted GOD in all things. Because He is in control, Patty's words of wisdom gave me confidence.

While listening to Patty on Oprah, something happened in my mind: I saw everything in a different light. At that moment, I knew that GOD was real, and that he wanted me to know that he loved me, and that there was more to life for me than being in the state that I was in. I was turning into a bald-headed paranoid drunk, but GOD had opened my eyes and I saw what I was doing to myself. I realized that I had just given up on life, and I knew that I had to go back to what Mama tried to teach me. I had to put my faith in GOD to get those thoughts out of my head, and to know that I had a lot of reasons to stick around and live.

I thank GOD for the Oprah show. I got more from her show that day than entertainment: what I got was a message that kept me alive. I kept my doctor's appointment that day because Chris went through the trouble of making it for me when I needed it. I'd had an encounter with GOD that day that I still can't explain. I knew for sure that He loved me, and He wanted me to get it together. Now, I thank GOD for every birthday I have, and that He continues to wake me up each morning, to surround me with His love, and keep me with a sound mind and body. I stayed in Charlotte for a while, and got myself together. I began calling the family back home. Then I prepared myself to go back Miami, Florida.

CHAPTER FIVE

BACK IN MIAMI, JUNE 1998

When I returned to Miami, Daddy had retired. He and Mama had been taking trips to visit their families. They went to Tallahassee and Tampa. They even went to New York to see Daddy's brothers. As he told me about their trip, I noticed that Mama had nothing to say. Mama always had something funny to say about Daddy's brothers, but she was silent. I asked Mama how she liked her vacation, but she did not respond the way I thought she should have, she just sat there looking out the screen door.

Mama seemed to be distracted by something outside. I stood up to see what she was looking at, but there was nothing going on outside that should have taken her attention away from our conversation.

Daddy could see that I was concerned about Mama's behavior but he kept on talking about their trip. While Daddy was still talking about their vacation, I couldn't help but cut him off to talk to Mama.

"What's wrong, Mama?" I asked, but before she could answer me, Daddy said Mama needed to get some rest. It was as if he didn't want me to notice the change in Mama, so he wanted to get her out of the room.

"Who, me?" Mama answered ten minutes later. Mama's response was very slow.

I thought it was rude of Daddy to interrupt our conversation while I was still talking to Mama, but I didn't say anything because he's weird like that sometimes.

"Your Mama's tired. We had a long day today," Daddy said.

Daddy made excuses for Mama's new personality. He had an idea that something was wrong even then, but he didn't want to admit it. When Bobbie was killed, I had a hard time dealing with my sister's death. It had to be even harder for Mama. I can't even imagine how it might feel to lose one of my children. "Mama may have had a serious case of emptiness," I thought. A lot had happened in the past few years and no one knows how much one person can take. I still felt that something was wrong with Mama.

I'd come home and hoped that everyone was able to move on. But somehow an unexpected storm had hit our family and was blowing it apart, piece by piece. The death of my sisters and Mama's new personality had come along and upset our sound and grounded family life.

Our family seemed to be dysfunctional. Mama had been the cornerstone of our family's foundation. She was the one person everyone counted on to keep it together. Sometimes, I'd cry myself to sleep at night because I didn't like what was happening to our family. Something was wrong with Mama, but everyone turned their heads and acted as if there was no problem, and I was just as guilty but not for long.

At first, I thought Mama was going into a deep depression, but after a while, it occurred to me that Mama could be developing Alzheimer's. I kept putting the thought out of my head, but Mama wasn't herself anymore; she kept doing and saying things that were out of character for her. She was slipping away from me and there was nothing I could do about it.

Mama was becoming a stranger to me. It still took some time for me to admit to myself that she might have Alzheimer's.

The thought was too painful for me to think about; I couldn't even say it out loud to myself, because admitting it would make it a reality that I didn't want to accept. The only thing I had to hang on to was that from what I could see, she still looked like Mama. But when I really looked into her eyes, Mama wasn't in there.

Out of all of the drama that was going on, the family still managed to hold on and communicate with each other.

I was in search of a more meaningful spiritual life. I asked GOD to help me change my lifestyle. I began to read my Bible and meditate for a while. I wanted to keep negative thoughts out of my mind. When I got back to Miami, I remembered that I had given everything away except my personal belongings before I left. And they were still in storage. I had not found a place of my own to live yet, but I had talked to my best friend, Sandra, before I left Charlotte. She invited me to stay with her for as long as I needed to. Sandra had a big heart; I've always adored our friendship. Sandra and I went to high school together. We had been friends for at least thirty years.

There was no one living at home but Mama and Dad when I got back from Charlotte. Daddy had set new house rules since we'd all left home and had our own families. He said that his doors were closed and locked, and the lights were out at six o'clock. That wasn't quite the schedule I'd plan to keep, so with all respect to Daddy's wishes, I was better off at Sandra's house, I thought.

Daddy said that the neighborhood had changed and he was right: Everything was different. When I was growing up there, the neighborhood was nice and safe. You could even walk to the park and sit on the park benches and talk, or just enjoy the weather without looking over your shoulder after dark. People died of natural causes, not robberies.

Daddy said if anyone came into his yard after six, they'd have to answer to him. No one bothered visiting them after six, because we didn't want Daddy to get excited enough to try pulling that old gun that he always talked about out of the closet.

Sandra only lived a few blocks from their house, so I was in walking distance and was able to keep an eye on Mama.

Sandra was a hard worker, she was dedicated, and a responsible person, but Sandra was also a party girl. I was trying to change my lifestyle; I felt that I should be doing something else with my life.

Kena, my youngest daughter, had gotten married and had her own family. I was suddenly left with nothing to do, and no one to care for. I wished I could talk to Mama, she always knew what to do, but if I had guessed right about her having Alzheimer's, Mama would soon need someone to tell her what to do. I felt a void in my life, but I didn't know what I needed to fill it.

Sandra was my best friend and she wanted to show me how much everyone had missed me, so she wanted to celebrate my return to Miami (and every weekend, it seemed). I found myself trying to party with the crowd again, but it didn't satisfy me anymore, not the way it had before; something was missing and I didn't know what it was. I was also worried about Mama's personality changes. Something had happened to her and it was upsetting everything and everyone around her; I was really concerned.

I had not seen Mama in a couple of days. I was still staying with Sandra. She was at work and I had been offered a job that I would began in a week. I was so excited about the good news, I wanted to tell anyone that would listen about my news. I wanted to let them know that I had taken a private duty case in Coral Gables, and I'd only see them on the weekends. I took a walk around the corner to visit Mama, and to let her and Dad know when I'd start working. When I got there, Mama was dressed a little strangely: She had on several layers of winter clothing. Nothing matched, or should have even been worn on such a hot and humid day. This was a sign that something was wrong with Mama. How was I going to handle it?

When I walked into the house, it was a wreck. Daddy never did do anything around the house before Mama got sick, because she had to pick up after him. It was up to Daddy to pick up things around the house, because Mama didn't seem to care anymore.

"Oh! I didn't know we were going to have company today, or I would have picked up the house a little bit," Daddy said as he let me into the house. I smiled and I thought, "Yeah, right! When did you ever clean up?" Before Mama got sick, she always kept things neat and clean and in perfect order.

We walked back to the dining room table where they were sitting when I came in. They were eating from take-out food containers. I sat at the table with them to talk and to find out how Mama was doing.

"Hey, Mama, you're not cooking today?" I asked.

I stacked the open mail into a pile and pushed the old food containers to the side. They looked like they'd been sitting there from the day before, and some of the containers still had food in them.

But Daddy answered instead of Mama.

"I told your mama that I don't think she ought to be cooking anymore. She act like she forgot what to do in the kitchen."

"What do you mean, Daddy?"

"Yesterday, she must have wanted to cook something and she turned all of the knobs on the stove on high, then she went into the living room and sat down to watch a movie on TV. She could have burned the house down. Anyway, I went to Sadie's to order us some dinner, and look, she's hardly eaten a thing."

Mama stopped eating and stared at Daddy. He looked at her and smiled. Mama rolled her eyes at him. Daddy looked at me, and opened his take-out container and finished his lunch.

"What's that old man talking about?" Mama asked as she rolled her eyes at Daddy again. She pushed the take-out container that she was eating from to the side, and almost on the floor. Mama started to cry.

"What's wrong, Mama? Are you in pain?"

I got up and went over to comfort her.

"Hell no! I'm not in pain! I just want my money back!" Mama began to look into her purse and inside of her bra for her money. Mama always kept money in her bra; she said it was her "personal bank." She put money on the left side, all other valuables on the right side. But Mama didn't find the money that she was looking for.

"What money, Mama? When did you lose it?" I took the purse from Mama and sat down next to her, I began to look in the purse to see if she had overlooked it. But Mama snatched the purse out of my hands and accused me of trying to steal her money.

"Robert is always stealing my money, and now you are, too." I was shocked at Mama's hostility and accusations. "Where is this all coming from?" I thought.

When I looked at Daddy, I could see that he was very angry. His nose had turned red and frowns were in his forehead. I knew then that things were getting serious and out of hand.

"Daddy! What's Mama talking about?" I asked as I stood between both of them.

"I don't talk to that woman when she starts talking crazy," Daddy said, as he got up from the table and stormed into their bedroom.

Mama stood up with her walker and went into the living room to sit in her La-z-boy chair. Once Mama was seated in the chair, she began to cry again.

"Mama, please don't cry...just tell me what's going on," I said, but Mama just waved me away.

I didn't want to pressure her for an answer at the moment. I was headed into their bedroom where Daddy had gone to see what was going on, but Mama called me back before I got there. Forgetting that she'd just waved me away and out of her face just a moment ago, she said, "Where are you going, girl? I'm trying to tell you what happened and you're walking away. He steals my money all of the time," Mama said as she shook her finger in the direction of their room where Daddy had gone.

"What makes you think that he's stealing your money, Mama?" I asked.

"When we go to the bank, I always have the bank lady to give me 100 dollars in twenty-dollar bills, and she always put it in an envelope for me. I always put the money into my top drawer, and the next day, it's gone.

Mama sounded like she knew what she was talking about, I thought. That's what always threw me off about Mama.

Sometimes she's her old self, and then some days she's confused. But I'd have to check it out with Daddy because sometimes Mama had trouble remembering what happened.

"Mama, why are you withdrawing so much?" I asked. "I'm sure you don't need to withdraw that much money every time you go to the bank."

"Damn it, girl, it's my money, and I can take out as much as I want. How in the hell do you know how much I need?"

Mama had never talk to me with such hostility before.

"Mama, what's wrong? Why are you so angry?" I asked. I then realized at that moment that what I had suspected early on was now a sure reality: Mama was developing Alzheimer's.

I could hear Daddy calling me from his room, but someone was knocking at the door. I went to the door to see who was knocking. When I opened the door, a crack addict appeared, I thought, but when I looked closer, I saw that it was Daveon, the neighborhood drunk.

Daveon was about fifty years old now. He graduated from high school with my sister, and went into the military. When he got out, he got married and he and his wife had a son. Daveon said the stress of a family was too much, so his wife divorced him, and he moved back home with his mother. He's been there ever since.

I was concerned about Daveon coming in and out of our house if he was also on drugs, so I asked him, "Daveon, are you on drugs?"

He made a face as if he was insulted, then he smiled and said, "Not really — only when I can afford it."

I shook my head and I thought, "I'll have to keep my eye on him."

Daveon used to be a good-looking guy who had just four good teeth in the top of his mouth, skip a few and two in the bottom that are all the wrong colors, he'll show them off when he offers his wide smile. Daveon folded his bony arms across his chest and tried to start a conversation that I didn't have time for. Then Daddy came out of his room and called out to Daveon.

"Daveon, wait a minute; I've got a job for you."

I didn't want to talk to Daddy about anything while Daveon was standing there reeking of booze and tobacco, so I tried to get rid of him before Daddy got to the porch, but I was too late. Daddy hurried out to the porch and told Daveon that he had some handiwork for him to do. Daveon always looked for odd jobs around the neighborhood to earn money to buy his booze.

I asked Mama if she was all right and she said that she was. Her tears were gone and she'd forgotten all about the money she had accused Daddy of stealing. But I still needed some answers. I needed to know what was going on. Mama stopped crying and she began to watch the TV. Daddy was still talking to Daveon, and I seemed to be the only one still upset about what had just taken place in the dining room.

I cleaned the kitchen, the living room, and the bathroom, and made their beds. When Daddy finished talking to Daveon, he told me to follow him and I did. He went back into his room and opened up the chest of drawers and pointed to six envelopes. They were all from the same bank, and they all had 100 dollars in them.

Then Daddy said, "Lately, every time that woman go to the bank with me, she withdraws $100.00, and she don't even need it. I pay the bills and buy food, from my social security check. As soon as we leave the bank and get back home, I'll watch the TV while she's in and out of the rooms opening the drawers for the rest of the day hiding her money, and then moving it from one place to the other, until she forgets where she put it last.

"Whenever I find the money and give it back to her, she says I stole it from her. I don't want to fight, so I start putting it in this drawer."

Looking down into the drawer I could see six thick bank envelopes. "So Mama have her own separate checking account now?"

"Your Mama opened her own checking account the day she got her first social security check."

I smiled and I thought to myself, "You GO, Mom!" (because Daddy always controlled the money).

"I think we need to do something about this, Daddy," I said.

"Now, I don't want y'all to go to that bank telling them folks nothing about your mama, cause they might think she's crazy or something."

"What about you, Daddy? Do you think she's crazy?"

"NO! I don't think my wife is crazy," he yelled loudly, with a wild look in his eyes.

"SHHH! Don't talk so loud, Daddy; she'll hear you," I cautioned him.

"Oh! Now you don't want your Mama to know that you said she's crazy."

"I didn't say that, Daddy, but if you don't think she's crazy, neither will the bank tellers."

Even though I tried to make myself clear to Daddy, he only heard what he wanted to hear. And when I hear that conversation again, I'll hear one of my sisters say, "Daddy says you think Mama is crazy." (But we'll laugh about it because they already know that he has selective hearing.)

Daddy and I agreed that he should just deposit the money back into Mama's account. We would later have to have papers drawn up so that my sisters and I could make medical and financial decisions for Mama in case something happened to Daddy. Before then, he was in charge of everything at the time, but Mama was not able to conduct her own business.

When I got back to Sandra's house, I called my sisters and told them my concerns. Clara said that she'd watch them much closer now that she knew what was going on.

It got harder to visit Mama, even though we knew we should. You never knew what kind of mood Mama was going to be in. You never knew when she was going to curse you out or act as if you were an intruder.

We laughed at some of the things Mama did and said, but Alzheimer's was never seriously discussed among my sisters and me (but it was always in the back of my mind).

There was a time when Mama was making some wild accusations about a few things: Mama accused my sister Karen of stealing her canned goods from the cupboard, and she said that one of her new neighbors came in and stole the hot sauce from the dining room table.

I told my sisters Clara and Karen that it's important that we keep going over to see them (even though it takes a lot of strength to visit them when you know you'll be greeted with anger, or when you know the person you love might call you names or even accuse you of stealing from her). "We need to give Mama a chance to express her anger," I thought, "and maybe if we kept being there for her — no matter what — she wouldn't be so hostile."

With Alzheimer's sufferers, you just love them as they are.

CHAPTER SIX

(AUGUST 1998)
WORKING FOR MR. HEINZ

When I started working for Mr. Heinz, he was a very sick man. He was eighty-seven years old. He'd had a stroke and was unable to move his right arm and leg. He was a little German guy, about five feet three and he weighed maybe a hundred pounds. His wife had died several years earlier, but in her childbearing years, Mrs. Heinz was never able to have children.

As they got on in years, Mr. Heinz had an affair with a younger woman. His infidelity led to the birth of his daughter, Marene. Mr. Heinz was a millionaire. He paid a lawyer to help him get sole custody of Marene when she was an infant. He and his wife raised and educated her until she was a grown-up young lady and moved out. Mr. Heinz's wife died before Marene finished college. Despite the loss of her mother, she continued her education and later moved to Colorado.

When I took Mr. Heinz's private duty case, they didn't expect him to be around very long. I was told that the assignment would only last for six or eight weeks. He was a weak, pale, and skinny little man who only spoke above a whisper. But with lots of care, attention, and understanding, the good LORD helped me to keep him around a few more years.

Once Mr. Heinz's health improved and he'd gain at least ten pounds, he was ready to see his old friends again. Mr. Heinz had me call a few of his special friends to come over to visit. When one of his "special friends" came to visit, I was surprised to see a fifty-year-old blonde female with a dark tan who drove up to the front gate in a beautiful black BMW. I buzzed her in and watched her from the huge window in the TV room, as she pulled up and parked in the driveway in front of the house. She got out and walked up the steps to the porch, and I met her at the front door and let her in.

She smiled and told me that her name was Cherlyn. She spoke with a high-pitched voice, and she whined when she talked. After we greeted each other, she walked over to Mr. Heinz and sat in the chair next to him. She leaned over and kissed him on the mouth, which seemed longer than I thought she ought to. It had not been that long since Mr. Heinz had strength enough to even sit up by himself, and I didn't want her to hurt him.

Cherlyn cried and hugged Mr. Heinz, pulling him into her well-endowed chest. His smile was wide enough to make his eyes close as his head sank into her two puffy pillows.

I thought to myself, "Please, let him up for air! I've worked hard to bring him this far, don't kill him now," but instead, I jokingly said, "All right! Cherlyn, don't get him too excited!" We all laughed and agreed that she should back off a little.

Mr. Heinz was smiling as he pulled Cherlyn's hand to his face. Then he looked up and told me that she was his girlfriend.

"What a couple!" I thought. "An eighty-seven-year-old senior citizen, dating a middle-aged blonde." They had been together for eight years and his daughter, Marene, hated Cherlyn.

When Mr. Heinz had an affair with the younger woman (who, by the way, was not Cherlyn) he was sixty years old. Marene was twenty-seven years old when I met her.

Before Mr. Heinz got sick, he bought Cherlyn a new house and a new car. (The house she already had was destroyed by Hurricane Andrew.) Her car was also totaled when the trees and debris that were uprooted were tossed about.

The house and the car that Mr. Heinz bought for Cherlyn had been paid for already. Cherlyn said that he'd paid for her to live in a deluxe apartment for four years and then bought her a new house, and another car. He promised her that after three years, she could not only have the titles to the car and the deeds to the house, she could have another new car.

Three years and a few months had passed already and Cherlyn had come by the house to go out to dinner with Mr. Heinz and to celebrate her getting the documents, and to look at some new cars. She didn't know that Marene had come home to visit her father. When Marene learned of what they were celebrating, she and Cherlyn had a terrible fight about Cherlyn taking advantage of her father.

During the fight, Mr. Heinz got very excited. He had a stroke and a heart attack and was hospitalized for several months.

Cherlyn was not permitted to visit Mr. Heinz, at his daughter's request. Cherlyn got an attorney to protest Marene's request. Mr. Heinz's case went to probate court; his daughter wanted to declare him incompetent.

One of the most brilliant probate attorneys in Coral Gables, Florida took the case: Ms. Joyce Karr, of Karr and Karr. Mr. Heinz's health took a turn for the worst and his daughter wanted to return to Colorado after she learned that the courts had appointed Ms. Karr to be his medical and financial power of attorney.

"Who is Joyce Karr?" she asked when she called me for information on the case.

Before Marene went back to Colorado, she watched me work with her father. When she saw how well he responded to my care, she made a few phone calls of her own. She soon realized that Joyce Karr had hired one of the best certified caregivers in Miami.

Even though the relationship between Marene and her father was a little cold and distant, she still wanted to know that he was being well taken care of and was in good hands.

When Marene went back to Colorado, Cherlyn and I became very good friends. She got permission from Joyce Karr and the courts to visit with Mr. Heinz again. She came over at least three or four times a week. We went shopping at Dade Land Mall, or Sawgrass Mills; we had lunch and dinner at the best of restaurants (or wherever Cherlyn wanted to go). We even visited the printing factory that Mr. Heinz once owned.

Before Mr. Heinz had the stroke, Cherlyn said that he was a very active man, and they had a lot of fun together. Mr. Heinz was in a wheelchair after his stroke. Whenever we'd go somewhere, I'd get him in and out of the front seat of the car. Cherlyn would drive and I'd sit in back. When we'd stop, I'd get Mr. Heinz out of the car and into his wheelchair, and Cherlyn would push him around the mall and wherever we went. When she pushed him in the wheelchair, or while he sat in the front seat with Cherlyn, she often called him Fritz, which was his first name, and he'd call her "his little nibbling" as she kissed him, rubbed his head and chest. All the while, he blushed and smiled. Cherlyn seemed to pour a lot of life into Mr. Heinz whenever she was around.

It was Christmas time, and Mr. Heinz's daughter had come back home to visit him for the holidays. Cherlyn had stopped by the house one evening to drop off some gifts, but she didn't know that his daughter had come home to visit. Marene went into a rage; she said that Cherlyn had come over too late. She said that it was after nine at night and that Cherlyn was being disrespectful for coming by that late. They had another fight. They were two blonde-headed, blue-eyed women who hated each other.

When Cherlyn left the house that night, we didn't hear from her for several days. She didn't even come or call for Christmas. Mr. Heinz wanted me to get in touch with her. I tried to reach her several times by phone, but I never got an answer. Mr. Heinz's Christmas was ruined, and all of Cherlyn's gifts were still under the Christmas tree waiting for her to open them.

Mr. Heinz was very agitated and displeased with his daughter. After visiting for a week, Marene was back in Colorado by New Year's Eve. Several weeks had passed, and we still had not heard from Cherlyn. I tried calling her but I got no answer. Mr. Heinz was even more agitated and nothing pleased him. As the days passed, Mr. Heinz began having memory lapses. At the times he thought that he was someplace else, and not in his own home, he made me think about Mama and her episodes.

Mr. Heinz was older than Mama, but her dementia had been a little more advanced than his (although I wasn't too sure at that point whose was worse). Mr. Heinz memory was disappearing, and so was the once-vibrant, energetic, little man I had grown to know.

Mr. Heinz owned a printing press factory, and he'd also invented some type of hair curler when he lived in Argentina. He was a retired millionaire. Mr. Heinz often got confused with living in the moment and living in the past. One morning after I helped him get dressed, and served him breakfast, he said he wanted to go by the factory. I'd been there with him when Cherlyn was still coming around. Everyone loved him there; they all called him "Mr. Fritz," and they made him feel wanted and loved. I wished I'd been able to contact Cherlyn that morning.

When Mr. Heinz finished his breakfast, I put him into his wheelchair and then into his grey Mercedes-Benz. Off we went to Hialeah (where the factory was); he told me to hurry up and park because we were running late, and he had things to do inside.

Once we got inside, he wanted to go to the main office. I thought he wanted to greet and talk to some of the managers, but that wasn't the case. Mr. Heinz thought that he had come in to work, and it was business as usual. He'd forgotten that he'd sold the company and was retired. He began to order everyone around and asked questions about the new help.

Once I realized what was happening with him, I bid everyone good morning for both of us and I rolled him out of the office and then out of the building. He cursed me and fussed at me all the way to the car. When we got to the car, Mr. Heinz wanted to drive back home. I spent almost an hour trying to talk him into letting me help him into the car and letting me drive home. Mr. Heinz cursed me all the way back to his house. When we got into the house, I gave him lunch and something to settle him down.

The next day was Saturday. Joyce had hired someone to relieve me on the weekends. I called home to see how Mama was doing, and to let Daddy know that I'd be home the next day. I also called Sandra to let her know that I was off for the weekend. She said she was having another party that weekend, and she had a surprise for me.

CHAPTER SEVEN

HOME FOR THE WEEKEND

My first stop was home; I had to see Mama. I'd talked to her on the phone but sometimes Mama didn't make much sense when you talked to her. I needed to see her in person.

Daddy had told me that the neurologist wanted to see Mama in his office, and I had to get all of the details. While I was there, Mama wanted me to stay a little longer. I called Sandra to let her know that I was going to spend the entire day with Mama, and I'd see her later that evening. I spent the rest of the day with Mama, although she had mood swings. Sometimes, she had trouble remembering things she had said or requests she had made (such as, an hour after she'd asked me to stay with her, she wanted to know why was I still hanging around her house). I never took Mama seriously anymore; once I'd caught on to how her mind clicked on and off, it became easy to take her insults; she was funny.

Around six o'clock, I called Sandra. Her phone rang, and when she answered it, the music was so loud I could hardly hear her. Once she turned the music down, I could hear a familiar voice in the background, I recognized the Bahamian accent and I knew it was Balie. Sandra's voice came in nice and clear, "Okay, Ellen, come whenever you are ready, but hold on — someone wants to talk to you," she yelled, still having to talk above the music.

"Sandra! Wait!" I shouted. My first reaction was to hang up the phone, but I decided against it.

Balie was a personal friend of mine. In fact, we were dating before I lost my head and moved to Charlotte. When I left, I didn't even tell him that I was going or why I was leaving. While I was in Charlotte, he sent messages by Sandra, at least two or three times a week, asking me to call and talk to him. I told Sandra I didn't want to hear from him again.

"Hello, Ellen. Are you all right?" Balie asked.

"Yes, I'm fine."

I cleared my throat while I tried to think of something to say. It was hard to talk with Mama standing on her walker right in front of me, smiling and looking right into my mouth every time I opened it. She was so close, I could feel her breathing my air. Daddy was sitting down in the chair next to the phone waiting to hear the rest of my conversation. I was ready to get out of there.

When I put the phone closer to my ear, I could hear Balie saying to me, "I just wanted to hear your voice, and I also wanted to say that I still love you."

I closed my eyes and took a deep breath. The weight of Balie's words wooed me, his smooth voice made me remember all the feelings I had for him before I went to Charlotte.

Balie was a sixty-year-old Bahamian man whose body was in better shape that most forty-year-olds. We always found ourselves deeply involved in interesting conversations, or laughing about some story he'd made up. I was ready to get out of the house; it felt like Mom and Dad were suffocating me. I had to rush Balie off of the phone, and get Mama settled in for the night.

"Okay, Balie, I'm going to help my mom get ready for bed and I'll see you later." I had to make myself snap back; his voice was making me have feelings I didn't want to feel.

I pointed toward Mama's room and she turned her walker in that direction. She had been hanging on to my every word while I was on the phone. It was already after six o'clock and Daddy was ready to shut it down. I helped Mama get ready for bed and I left.

When I drove up to Sandra's house, every single light in her house seemed to be turned on. The yard was already filled with cars, and it looked like they'd started early. I drove a block down the street, parked, and walked backed to the house. As I walked back to Sandra's house, I hoped that someone was near the door when I knocked. I didn't have a key, and the music was so loud if no one heard me knocking, I could have been standing outside forever.

When I knocked, the door opened right away, and Balie's chocolate face appeared. I checked him out and he still looked good. He had on khaki Dockers, a blue polo shirt, brown loafers, and a sexy smile. He kissed me on the cheek, took my hand, and pulled me into the crowded house.

"Lets get a drink," Balie offered, as he put both hands on my shoulders and walked in back of me as he guided me through the crowd toward the kitchen. Balie followed me very closely (so closely I could feel him breathing on my neck). Balie was a smooth old dude, and I could tell what was on his mind by the gestures that he made, but he had a rude awakening coming. All I had time for was a drink together and a little conversation.

If I had my own place, I wouldn't even have been there, but I lived there on the weekend, so I had no choice. But I was going to make sure that would change. We got our drinks and found a little cozy spot in a corner so we could talk and catch up on each other's lives. I confessed my irresponsible actions to Balie and said that I was sorry. Then I told him that I really didn't want to rekindle the intimate relationship that we had before I left. I said, "Balie, I still care about you, but I only want to be friends. I hope you agree. Please don't argue with me. "

"You can't really mean that, Ellen. I know you still love me; I can see it in your eyes."

Balie leaned over to me, and he talked right into my face. He was so close, I could feel his lips brush against my cheek.

A little closer and he could have kissed me. I almost wanted him to. Balie had that kind of effect on me. I still loved him but there was no real passion between us anymore, not as there had been before. I had come to the realization that although I found Balie very charming, it was too late for us intimately. I needed time to find out what was happening to me. I pushed him away from me and put my drink to my lips.

"I'm sure you didn't just put your life on hold all of this time, just waiting for me to come back," I said. I was already feeling guilty that I had not handled the situation the way I should have. Then hearing Balie say that he still loved me made me feel worse.

"No, I didn't just sit around and wait, but I did wonder why you never wrote or even called."

"I said that I was sorry, Balie; what more do you want from my life?" I snapped.

Balie lived in Nassau; he owned a fishing business there, but every month, he'd fly into Miami at least one day ahead of his crew. Once they'd docked, he'd do his business with the fish market merchants on the water front. When ever he was in Miami, he'd stay two or three days after he'd finished with his business and he'd hang out with me for a few days, and then go back to Nassau, which was fine with me. I loved Balie very much at the time, but I was glad that he was only a distant lover. He needed a lot of attention, and I was entering menopause and anything else would have been too much for me to handle. Between the hot flashes and the mood swings, Balie was always lucky enough to catch me on the days when my hormones weren't jumping all over the place. When I returned from Charlotte, I was in search of something different in my life. I didn't know what it was, but I knew that it wasn't the kind of life I had before, and I also knew it didn't include Balie.

There was silence between us. And I thought to myself, "Thanks for understanding, Balie."

Balie took the glass out of my hand and sat it on the table.

"Listen, Ellen, couldn't we just have this last night together in each other's arms?"

"No, he didn't say that!" I thought. Balie had pissed me off.

What did Balie think? That we'd just have one last hoorah, and go our separate ways? I shook my head and gave him a look that made him stand up.

"Look, Balie, why don't you just take a walk," I said.

I thought to myself, "Why couldn't he just let it go?" I was already consumed with issues from my past, I needed time to myself.

Balie picked up his drink, and headed toward the bar in Sandra's kitchen. My eyes followed him as I sat on the couch, still pouting. Through the crowd I could see him talking to Sandra; they were looking in my direction. Before I could react, Rita sat on the couch next to me. She had been listening to my conversation with Balie. Rita was the type of person who couldn't take a hint, even if you put it in her hand.

Her hair was braided in what looked like a thousand braids; it seemed to be too much for a woman her age, and her outfit was far from conservative. Her perfectly drawn eyebrows, and her scandalously red lipstick jumped right out at me, as she slid down in the seat next to me.

"Ellen, I couldn't help but hear the way you brushed Balie off," she said in a low voice.

Rita and I were never that close, and now she had the nerve to listen to my conversation and then comment on it? I didn't want to talk to Rita at that moment; my focus was on Balie and Sandra talking together and looking at me from across the room. Rita was lucky I was trying to change my lifestyle, or I would have read Rita from A to Z. But I wouldn't even respond to Rita's comment. I didn't even want to acknowledge the fact that she was even sitting there, but my manners wouldn't let me be so rude.

"Oh, hi, Rita, how's it going?" I said. Rita patted me on the shoulder and gave me a look of sympathy.

"You're probably still upset over your sister's death," she said, "Sandra told me how it affected you, leaving town and everything, you didn't even tell the man what was going on."

At that moment, my blood pressure must have hit 2000. "EXCUSE ME!" I said harshly. "But why are you talking to me about MY personal business?" My words were quick and snappy.

I looked around for another seat, but they were all taken. I finished the rest of my drink, looked at my watch, and tried to keep my composure. I turned my attention to someone dancing on the floor to keep from choking Rita.

"Okay, Ellen, I'm not going to say another word about Balie. I just thought that you shouldn't be so hard on him. I always thought you two were a great couple."

If Rita would have said one more thing about me and Balie, I didn't know if I could have controlled myself.

"Well, I'm not going to give Balie another chance, and if you want him, then he's all yours." I looked at Rita, letting her know that her presence was not desired.

Rita laughed at my anger, and got on another subject.

"So! Are you still reading the Good Book?" Rita called the Bible "the Good Book."

I kept thinking to myself, "Why don't she just go away? Can't she see that I don't want to talk to her?" I was in a cozy little spot away from most of the noise, and Rita had invaded my space. I hoped she'd leave.

"Yeah, Rita, I'm still reading the Bible," I answered, letting her know I was annoyed with her sitting there.

"Sandra said that you wanted to change your lifestyle, but you know she's not going to let you do that! Shoot, Sandra is a party animal."

"I know," I answered, as I looked around the room trying hard not to pay attention to what Rita was saying.

"OH NO!" Rita blurted out. "It's happening to you already! That's why I don't mess with it, when you start messin' around with that Good Book, something happens to you — you're going to lose your mind," She blurted out again.

"Rita's such a fool," I thought to myself, "What's she talking about now?"

"What are you talking about, Rita? What's happening to me?"

"Your attitude, Ellen! Look at the way you're acting! You don't even know how to have a good time anymore! You're not even enjoying this party tonight, are you? If you don't straighten up soon, nobody is going to want to be around you while you're reading that stuff," she informed me.

"Rita, does it look like I care if no one wants to be around me?" I said in a sarcastic tone. I stared at Rita and folded my arms in front of me.

"You will when no one wants to talk to you," Rita said.

Taking another drink, Rita began to look around, her glance wondered around the room and then came back to me.

"And where is all of this knowledge coming from, Rita?" I said, letting my eyes wonder and looking in the ceiling.

"My sister in-law Janis started talking to her neighbor, who reads the Good Book. She gave one to Janis. Now I want you to know that Janis has lost her mind. She wants her husband, my brother, to stop doing things he's been doing for years."

"Like what, Rita?"

"Well, James does a few recreational drugs, and Janis used to do the same thing, but now, she's trying to act like she's better than my brother."

"Well, Rita, it wouldn't hurt for James to change his lifestyle, too."

"My brother says he's getting sick and tired of Janis and her mess. She won't even have a drink with him no more. "

Everyone in town knew that her whole family was on drugs, and that James Jr. and his father had a history of beating up their wives. Rita's brother, James, and his wife, Janis, both used to do all kind of drugs together. I'm sure that James's abusive behavior toward Janis while he was under the influence had a lot to do with Janis wanting to change their social habits. The beatings Janis endured made her want to stop indulging in what was causing her pain. Now that she doesn't want to indulge in it anymore, he wants to leave her.

"If James leaves Janis, it would be the best thing that could happen to her," I told Rita. I hoped everything worked out for her family, and that maybe James needed to read the Bible with Janis, or do something else, so that they'd have a common interest.

I couldn't believe that I was actually concerned about Rita's family enough to offer advice. But at the same time, I didn't want to hear anymore about her dysfunctional family either. So I got up and began to move around and mingle.

Once I began to mingle and greet my old friends, I found Sandra on the dance floor doing the electric slide. (This was a dance we loved in the '60s, but we had another name for it then.) Although we danced to other music, most of our music was from the '60s. We were all a generation of baby boomers who grew up in the '60s listening to Motown. You'd know it, too, by the music everyone danced to that night. We played music by the Temptations, Aretha, Smokey, and the Stylistics. No one there was under forty.

Sandra was waving her hand, motioning for me to come onto the floor and join them, but I shook my head no. I said that I'd sit that one out. I was waiting to talk to her about Balie, I wanted to know what they were talking about earlier, and why they were watching me when Rita sat down to talk to me.

When the music stopped, Sandra joined me. We sat at the dining room table and got caught up on what was going on. I found out that while I was in Charlotte, Baile had been dropping by Sandra's house on weekends when he was in town. Sandra said that a couple of times when Baile had dropped by, she was having a party. She said she invited him in and some of the girls, like Thelma and Rita started talking to Balie.

Sandra admitted that earlier that night, when they saw me talking to Rita when she sat on the couch next to me, Balie thought Rita was telling me about the affair she and Baile were having. Sandra said that they were watching to see what kind of a reaction I'd have once I knew about the affair. I realized that this was the reason they were watching me from across the room. I guess everyone in the house knew what had been going on (except me).

"Affair? What affair? How long has this been going on?" I asked.

I looked around the room for Rita. I was ready to slap her to sleep. Not for having an affair with Balie, but for having the nerve to sit in my face and talk trash about giving Balie another chance, when she knew all the time that she'd been sleeping with him.

"Hold up, Ellen — that happened after you told me that it was all over between you and Balie. Before Balie started coming here, Rita and Thelma and I all talked about how sad we felt for Balie. So he was fair game when they started at him."

"'Fair game?' she says? What does that mean?" I thought. "What kind of people have I been hanging out with? Is there no loyalty among friends anymore?"

"Why didn't you tell me what's been going on when I got back?"

"I had to see if you still felt the same about Balie. That's why I invited him here tonight. He'd called me yesterday to say he was in town. I told him that you would be here this weekend and that you two should talk. I wanted to give him a chance to tell you himself. He didn't, so that's why I'm telling you now."

Sandra poured me another drink but I pushed it away. I managed to control myself and I stopped looking for Rita. I decided to go to my bedroom, and on my way to my room, I could hear R. Kelly singing, "When a Woman's Fed Up." When I heard it, I stopped. Every time that song came on, all the females in the house would sing along with the record. Sandra called it "the national anthem for women."

I turned around to see who had put the CD in, and it was Balie. He motioned for me to come and dance with him. He looked like he'd had way too much to drink, but I walked back toward the dance floor. Balie thought I was coming back to dance with him, but I walked back to the table to ask Sandra if he was driving. But she'd already called his brother to pick him up. As I walked back to my room, I could hear Balie calling my name.

"Ellen! Dolling! Please dance with me." I'd always like Balie's Bahamian accent, but at that moment, I hated it. He didn't know that Sandra had told me about him and Rita. I waved him away and kept walking.

I went into my room and locked the door. I laid across my bed and closed my eyes, and when I opened them again, it was morning.

"Oh my goodness, it's morning already!" I shouted to myself.

I jumped up, took a shower, put on some clothes, and fixed my hair and makeup. All I needed was some coffee. I wanted to drop by to see how the folks were before I went back to work. When I walked to the front of the house, it looked as if a hurricane had blown through it.

As I cleaned up the cups, wine glasses, napkins, and paper plates, I couldn't help but think about the good times I'd had in that house with Balie. For a moment, my old feelings tried to rise to the top again. I closed my eyes and tried to picture us together, but I couldn't. I knew then that the thrill was gone. We could only be friends.

I hurried to finish cleaning up so I could leave, but I could hear Sandra's energetic and high-spirited footsteps moving toward the kitchen. The clinking of the wine glasses and serving dishes must have awakened her. I had a fresh pot of coffee brewing. We sat down and finished the conversation we'd started the night before.

"Ellen, Balie really cares about you, and if you feel the same about him, then you should reconsider and get back with him." Sandra's voice sounded sleepy as she took her first sip of coffee.

"I'm really not looking for a relationship with anyone now, Sandra," I said, "I need to be by myself for a while until I figure out what I want to do with the rest of my life."

Balie was the kind of man who seemed to need to have a woman in his life in some capacity wherever he went. I always knew that I wasn't really the only woman in Balie's life (although he never wanted to admit it). I didn't want to be the "other woman" in his life.

Sandra took a deep breath and another sip of coffee.

"You should think about spending the rest of your life with Balie. I think that's what he wants to do. He really don't want to be with Rita. He said that he's tried to break it off with her but she won't hear of it. Rita does everything but breathe for Balie."

Steam came from my ears every time I heard Rita's name.

"Well, she can have him. I told her that last night when she tried to give me advice on how to treat him."

I was sick of talking about Balie and Rita; it was only making me mad. I looked at my watch and I had not realized that so much time had passed in what seemed like such of a short amount of time. It was one o'clock already and the morning had disappeared.

I wanted to call Daddy but the phone rang before I could. Sandra picked it up and walked into her room, as she talked on the phone and sipped her coffee.

I was on my way to my room to get my purse, but someone knocked on the door. I went back to answer it. I opened the door and it was Balie, very neat and nicely dressed as always. He stood in the door way with six yellow roses in his hand. I stepped to the side to let him come in. Balie handed the roses to me.

"These are for you," he said. When Balie gave me the roses, he was smiling as if last night never happened. And all I could think about was him and Rita. I knew the roses were supposed to say, "I'm sorry and I want to get back with you again."

My head throbbed with anger and I felt like closing the door in his face, but I thought, "No; this will be the last time we'll see each other."

"Six roses? Not even a dozen?" I said, turning my lips up with disapproval.

"Six now and six when you say YES," Balie said. He reached into his pocket and pulled something out. But before he could finish talking, I began to blast him.

"Damn you, Balie! I told you last night!" I yelled.

But before I could finish talking, Balie took my hand and asked, "Ellen, will you marry me?"

He opened the little black velvet box and there was a beautiful diamond ring in it. His words sucked the breath right out of me, and I was almost blinded by the diamond ring. When I finally got my composure back, my mind was saying YES, but I could hear my mouth saying NO.

"No, Balie, I can't. I can't marry you."

His eyes and face were filled with disappointment. But the man who had just asked me to marry him had asked too late. I was not the same person who would have gladly said

"Yes!" before I went to Charlotte. Our lives had changed (or at least, mine had).

"Why not, Ellen? Why don't you want to marry me?"

"Balie, our lives have changed and too much has happened between us."

"You mean you're seeing someone else now?"

"The nerve of him, trying to be so innocent!" I thought.

"No, Balie, I mean you've been seeing Rita."

That was mean; I don't even know why I said that because Rita was not the reason I didn't want to marry Balie: It was just too late for us. I guess I just wanted him to feel guilty, so I wouldn't feel so bad about turning him down. Balie looked like he'd been caught with his hand in the cookie jar when I mentioned Rita's name.

"Oh, oh yeah, I've been talking to Rita while you were away."

"And that's it. You guys just talked?" I asked.

(No matter what Balie would have said, my answer still would have been no.)

"Okay, I have to confess, Ellen: I did take the woman out and we had a great time, but all we did was talk." I already knew the truth; Sandra had told me everything.

I'd given Balie a chance to come clean, even though it would not have changed anything, but he still lied, he lied until the end. I realized then that Balie was the type of man who'd only tell you what he thought you needed to know. I thought about what Mama had always told us about lying.

Mama said, "A half truth is still a whole lie." At that moment, I felt that everything between us had really diminished: There was no love, no desire, and no trust.

I asked Balie to leave.

Balie put the little velvet box back into his pocket, and I opened the front door and stood there until he walked out. As he passed by me, he stole a kiss from my cheek and walked out the door and got into his rented car. When Balie got into the car, he threw the other six yellow roses out of the window and pulled off. I watched his car grow smaller in the distance. I would never see him again.

I walked outside and picked up the roses. When I got back inside, Sandra was reading the card. Not knowing what had just happened, she read, "Six now and six when you say yes." Sandra read the card out loud and laid it on the table. She smiled as she looked at me. She was putting the yellow roses in a vase when I walked inside.

"I know, Sandra. That's what he told me when he gave them to me," I said.

Sandra grabbed my hand looking for the ring.

"Where is it? Where is the ring? Balie said he was going to give it to you this morning when he called from his cell phone. He was outside when he called. That's why I went into my room, he said he needed some privacy..." she rambled on.

But there was no ring.

Sandra sat down on the couch in front of the yellow roses that she had arranged so beautifully, and picked the card up again. She looked almost as disappointed as Balie had looked when I told him no.

"I didn't want the ring, Sandra! I said no."

"Ellen, you are a damn fool!" she yelled. Sandra got up, went back into her room, and closed the door.

Neither of us took each other's insults personally, but we'd always call each other on the B.S. In Sandra's mind, that's exactly what it was.

I was still holding dirty yellow roses that Balie had thrown out the window. I sat on the couch and picked out the baby's breath from the roses and put them into the vase with the others. I got up and called Daddy to let him know I was going to drop by before I went back to take care of Mr. Heinz.

I knocked on Sandra's room door; when she opened it, I told her that I was going to be moving. I offered to pay her for whatever she thought I should pay for staying there. I told her I wasn't mad; I just needed my own space.

I could see that Sandra was very upset that I wanted to move, but she got up anyway and gave me a hug. She said there was no charge, and no hard feelings, and that I should do whatever I thought was best for me.

I knew that things were going to be different. When I walked out that day, I was walking out of the only world I'd really known: a world of work, parties, and fun with my best friend. But I wanted more than that. I was headed for only God knows what.

When I got home, I could see Daddy standing on the screen porch. He opened the door as I emptied my trunk of all my belongings and put them into my room. I told Daddy that I'd be living at home on the weekends, whenever I was off, until I moved back into my own house, and he was very pleased.

After that crazy weekend at Sandra's house, I didn't know that it would be the last time that I'd get roses from a guy or the last time that I'd get a proposal of marriage. But getting married at that point and time was a variable I was not prepared for anyway. And if truth be told, I'm still okay with the answer that I gave Balie: I've learned to enjoy my own company, and I love being my own boss.

I later learned that Balie kept seeing Rita. They got back together, but Rita gave Balie the HIV virus. Rita died two years after they got together. Sometimes I think about Rita when I read my Bible; she was right. She said that when I start reading the Bible, it will change me. She said that I'd lose my mind. Rita was saying it in a negative way, but I thank GOD it did change me, and I'm glad that I lost the mind, because now I have the mind of Christ. The things I use to do no longer appeal to me anymore. It's like something has taken over my mind; I'm a different person now, but it's all good. I found out that GOD is what was missing in my life. And I thank him for finding me.

Balie doesn't visit or do business in Miami anymore; his son has taken over the business and dealings with merchants on a different level. They no longer get the personal service that Balie gave them. The last I heard, Balie was still living in Nassau, and he visits his brother in Miami occasionally. Sandra says that his once fine and healthy body has turned into that of a skinny old man.

CHAPTER EIGHT

MR. HEINZ'S BROKEN HEART

It was Sunday night when I got back to take care of Mr. Heinz. The caregiver who had relieved me said that Mr. Heinz had been calling my name the entire weekend. Mr. Heinz wouldn't eat, and he wouldn't even tell the caregiver when he had to use the bathroom, so the caregiver had diapers delivered to Mr. Heinz's home because he had become incontinent.

I stayed up with Mr. Heinz most of the night, hoping that I'd see some sign of saneness in his behavior by morning, but there was none. I called his daughter and I called Joyce Karr to notify them of his change in condition. During the next three or four weeks, Mr. Heinz had blood tests, an MRI, and some type of mental test that the doctor gave him in the office.

Mr. Heinz was in the first stages of the Alzheimer's. For me, Alzheimer's was everywhere it seemed: both at home with Mama, and now at work. Mr. Heinz was also being uncooperative and stubborn because he couldn't see Cherlyn. The last time his daughter had come to visit him, she had a fight with Cherlyn, and we had not seen or heard from her. I took Mr. Heinz out for lunch one day at a diner where he and Cherlyn loved to eat. I hoped that we'd run into her that day but we didn't. Kelly was our waitress; we always sat in her section whenever we'd eat at that diner.

When we were done eating, I asked Kelly to let Cherlyn know that Mr. Heinz was very sick and needed to see her. Kelly agreed that he looked bad, and she could see how the color seemed to have drained from his face. Mr. Heinz looked sickly and pale. Kelly said she wanted to help, and she'd give

Cherlyn the message when she came in to order deli meats for the week.

Two weeks later, Cherlyn came by the house, but by that time, Mr. Heinz seemed to have lost his will to live. He was in the bed and was not able to sit up anymore. Cherlyn began to visit him every day. Sometimes, she'd stay until midnight, talking to him and holding his hand. She even wanted to feed him his meals during the day. I told Cherlyn that it was okay with me for her to feed Mr. Heinz because he ate better when she fed him.

Within two weeks, Mr. Heinz was able to sit up by himself again, then he got strong enough to get into the wheelchair again, Cherlyn would push him around the house in the wheelchair while she talked to him. Sometimes, he'd remember who she was and sometimes, he'd just tell her to get the hell out.

Joyce Karr came over to visit a few times while Cherlyn was there. I made lunch for all of us, and Joyce observed Mr. Heinz's behavior, to see how far his dementia had advanced. She was satisfied that he was still able to enjoy the quality of life that he'd been used to.

"Mr. Heinz, do you have any summer plans yet?" Joyce asked.

He looked at Cherlyn and smiled as if he remembered the vacation they always enjoyed together.

"We're taking a cruise to the Bahamian Islands again," he answered. He and Cherlyn had just had the same conversation the day before. I was glad that Mr. Heinz was having a good day; he seemed sharper that day than he had in days past.

Cherlyn's face lit up. She talked about their summer cruise all the time. She'd already told me how she loved to play the slot machines. With the exception of the year that Mr. Heinz was in the hospital, he and Cherlyn had gone on a seven-day cruise In the Bahamas every summer every since she'd known him. Joyce said that she'd have to get the courts to release funds for Mr. Heinz, and that I should make arrangements for the three of us to go to the Bahamas together. They also used to take a trip to Palm Beach when they returned home from the cruise. I was very excited about the cruise and about the trip to Palm Beach for two weeks. I could hardly wait to get there.

But I was concerned about how Mr. Heinz would do on a cruise for seven days in his condition. Although Mr. Heinz had recovered better than I'd expected him to, he would still be away from the doctors that knew his medical history. If his doctors said that it was all right for him to go, who was I to worry?

The next week, we all went shopping and prepared for the cruise. Sometimes, Mr. Heinz had trouble remembering where we were or that we were even going on a cruise — or why we were even in the mall, for that matter — but Cherlyn reminded him and he was okay with whatever she said.

We finally went on the cruise. We played the slot machines, and the very first night, Cherlyn won $1,800 and I won $600. After I collected my winnings, I refused to play the slot machine anymore. Cherlyn lost everything she'd won the first time, but she occupied three of the slot machines most of the night and end up winning $3,000 in all.

The next day while Cherlyn kept Mr. Heinz busy, I had a chance to find my own space. I looked out over the beautiful waters and thought about what I wanted to do with the rest of my life, and how Mama's illness was going to affect me. I had accepted the fact that she had Alzheimer's, but I prayed that she wouldn't die and leave me. I didn't know if I could take it. I was getting depressed so I was glad that the high-pitched voice of Cherlyn — talking to Mr. Heinz getting closer to where I was standing it — interrupted my thoughts.

The cruise seemed to put Mr. Heinz more in touch with reality, and as long as he was in the range of Cherlyn's voice, he was okay. He laughed and smiled a lot. And even though his dementia didn't let him know what she was talking about sometimes, I was glad that he was happy again.

When we got back to Coral Gables, Cherlyn visited Mr. Heinz every day. His appetite was great, and the color had began to come back into his face.

We made plans to go to Palm Beach the next week. But Marene had come back to visit her father that same week. When she learned of our plans to go to Palm Beach, she wanted to go to with us. When Marene walked through the doors that day, I thought about our trip to Palm Beach and I knew we were going to have trouble.

Marene wanted to drive her father's car to Palm Beach, and Cherlyn wanted to drive her own car there. In an effort to keep Mr. Heinz from having another heart attack from the two of them fighting, I asked Cherlyn if she would please leave. Even though it I was Marene I really wanted to leave. In all of the confusion, Cherlyn refused to go on the trip with us.

Marene drove her father's car to Palm Beach, but he was very unhappy. He wouldn't even talk to her. We'd prepared to stay at a beautiful five-star hotel for two weeks, but after three days (during which Mr. Heinz refused to eat), we had to leave. I wanted to be near his doctors because he didn't look well.

On the ride back home to Coral Gables, no one talked the first fifty miles. Marene stopped to get some gas; when she got back into the car, she looked at her father and tried to talk to him.

"Dad, why do you hate me?" she said.

He did not answer her.

"Dad, I know that you're mad because SHE'S not here. Why?"

No answer.

"I don't know why you want to be around her — she only wants you for your money," Marene scolded her father.

Mr. Heinz looked at Marene like he really knew what she was saying to him. He raised his hand to hit her but he put it down. His sanity was really a reality at that moment, and he answered her in a loud and shaky voice.

"Do you think I've fooled myself into thinking that she wants me because I look so good?" he shouted.

Mr. Heinz started to cry.

"Look at me! I'm sick and crippled, and yet she talks to me and treats me as if I'm not. Can I at least spend my own money on something that makes me happy?"

He cried again.

Marene started to cry and so did I, but Mr. Heinz never spoke a single word after that day. Marene went back to Colorado, but she called at least twice a week to check on him.

Mr. Heinz lived at home for almost a year, after we'd returned from our trip to Palm Beach. After that year, he went into the hospital because he wouldn't eat, drink, or take his medications.

I called Marene and Joyce to let her know what was going on and Marene insisted that the doctors insert a feeding tube. Mr. Heinz lived with the feeding tube for about four weeks, and then he died. They said that Mr. Heinz died because he refused to eat, but I believe that Mr. Heinz really died of a broken heart.

Mr. Heinz lived in a beautiful 3 million-dollar home in Coral Gables, Florida. When he died, I had lived in it for almost two years. Marene didn't know what she wanted to do with the house on Palermo Drive. It was my residence for almost two years. I was being paid a generous salary to housesit and feed the cat. I didn't have the money of a millionaire, but I certainly lived like one. Marene wanted me to stay on much longer, but it was my decision to move out.

I had to snap back to reality and go back to work.

CHAPTER NINE

NEW EXPERIENCES

Mama seemed to be doing all right. Her dementia wasn't getting any worse and Daddy was still making all of her medical and financial decisions. I felt that I was not needed yet.

I moved out to Arizona when I got a call from Kena, who had moved from Beaufort, South Carolina to Luke Air Force Base, because her husband's orders transferred him there. She had asked me to spend some time with her in Arizona. Once I got to Arizona, I loved it. I applied for a job and I moved to Phoenix. Within months, I called Marene to let her know of my plans to move out West.

Once she got someone into the house, I moved out and went to Arizona. I worked there in a nursing home for a year. When my vacation time came around, I went back to Miami to check on Mama's condition. Sandra insisted that I stay at her house when I returned. This time around everything was very different.

My visit to Miami was not a pleasant one. Although my best friend Sandra had invited me to stay with her while I was in Miami, she was acting like a complete stranger. Mama was still losing weight. She had a very short attention span, and often forgot what she was saying in the middle of a conversation. I realized then that life at home would never be the same. My sisters and I had planned a family dinner for our mom and dad at their favorite restaurant. It was a family reunion dinner.

I went by the house to hurry them along. We were going to have dinner at six. It was my job to have them ready to go by five. Clara was going to drive us to the restaurant, and Karen went to the restaurant ahead of us to get enough tables (not too far from the bathroom, so Mama wouldn't have to walk too far when she had to go).

When I got to the house, I knocked, but no one answered. I knocked again. There was still no answer, so I then used my key to get in. As I opened the door, I still stood on the front porch. I didn't know what the mood was going to be when I got inside, so I yelled from the porch.

"HELLO! It's me, Ellen! I'm coming in."

"I know, I saw your car when you drove up," Daddy answered from the bedroom.

"Are you almost dressed?" I yelled back.

Mama answered this time, sounding very agitated.

"NO! We are not dressed yet and if you are ready to go, just leave."

"I just asked, Mama. Do you need any help?" Still standing in the living room, I started toward Mama's room, picking up pieces of clothing and shoes that had been left there because no one had bothered to clean.

"NO! I can dress myself!" Mama shouted back to me.

Mama used to be a very sharp dresser, but I was concerned about how she was going to look when she finished dressing for dinner that night. The last time I saw Mama dress herself to go out, she looked a little overdressed. I walked into their room while they were still dressing.

"Hey, Mama, that's a nice dress, but it looks like there is something on the front of it; let me help you find another dress," I offered. I was hoping that Mama would look down and realize that there were a few gravy stains that were very visible, and agree with me and take it off.

"You always trying to tell me what to do. I like this dress and I'm going to wear it tonight, or I'm not going."

I realized that I had used the wrong approach; Mama's dignity was threatened and she was still trying to stay in control. I worked with these types of patients all the time. I should known better, but it was hard for me to put Mama in the same category as some of the patients I'd taken care of. Knowing that Mama would soon be moving toward the middle and last stages of that horrible Alzheimer's disease someday was very painful.

Alzheimer's disease threatens the dignity of the sufferers. Mama was already aware that things were not right, and of things not being in her control anymore. It seemed like Mama could tell that I was being condescending or patronizing her.

Lashing out and not cooperating were her only ways of controlling the situation, and it looked like Mama was going to have the last word that evening.

I remembered that I had a sweater in the car that Mama loved.

I went back out to the car and got the sweater, and just as I was about to let myself back into the house with the key, my sister Clara drove up. I waited for her to get out of her car so that we could go into the house together. Daddy always got upset whenever he heard the doors opening and closing too much.

"Are they ready yet?" Clara asked. She was ready to go because she was running behind schedule.

"Almost. Mama has on a dress with gravy stains on the front of it, but she still want to wear it. I'm going to give her this sweater that she's always loved. When she puts it on, it will hide the gravy stains on her dress," I told her.

As we walked into the house, Lucy, Clara's adopted daughter, came running in the door.

"Is Grandma ready yet?" Lucy asked as she tried to catch her breath.

"Please! whatever you do, don't rush Mama, just wait in the living room until she's dressed."

We had to slow our pace down with Mama that night, and just shut out the usual rush of things. We had to just shift ourselves to the place that Mama was in, even if we did get to dinner late. We had to remind ourselves that Mama had always been there for us; now it was time for us to hang in there with her.

While we were at dinner, I found myself wanting to feed Mama or at least assist her, but she'd slap my hand and tell me to mind my own damn business. Everyone would laugh and tell me to relax.

Mom and Dad enjoyed their meal and were glad that we'd taken them out. When dinner was over, I walked with Mama to the bathroom, and the rest of them went to the car. Mama didn't want to go to the bathroom; she wanted to go with everyone else, but I knew that as soon as she got into the car, she'd have to go. I insisted that we go into the bathroom. Mama called me a few choice names, but I just laughed; I'd gotten used to the insults.

When Mama was done using the bathroom, we walked out to the front of the building and Clara pulled her car up so that we didn't have to walk that far. I helped Mama get in and Clara drove us back to the house and dropped us off. When we got inside, I helped Mama get out of her clothes. She told me to hang her dress up in the closet. I said okay but when Mama went into the bathroom, I put her dress in a small plastic bag and sat it near the door, so that I could take it with me to have it cleaned for her the next day. That must have been Mama's favorite dress. I'd buy her another one, or one just like it, but I didn't think they made that style of dress anymore.

I joined Daddy in the living room while he was watching the news on TV. We could hear Mama's walker on the wooden floor coming down the hall. Daddy yelled to her that we were sitting in the living room. But Mama said that she was going to bed. Daddy said that he'd finish watching the news in their room since Mama didn't want to sit up with him. Once they were in bed, I told them that I was going back to Arizona in a couple of days, but I'd see them before I left.

When I got to Arizona, I went back to work at the nursing home but I was depressed all of the time. I thought about Mama day and night. Should I go back? Should I try to get them to move to Phoenix? I didn't know what to do. Somehow, I'd convince myself that Mama would be all right, and I had to go on with my life, but everything in me was saying go home and take care of Mama.

CHAPTER TEN

SUNVIEW CARE CENTER

I began working at a nursing home in Youngtown, Arizona. I loved my job working as a caregiver at SunView Care Center, SunView Care Center was built in the middle of the Sun City retirement community. Many of the residents that lived in the community went for walks on the sidewalks and alleys around Sun View. Any of them could have easily been mistaken for one of the residents inside the building, which reminds me of an incident I must share with you

When I first got there, I worked on another unit. I was transferred to the Valencia Villa unit to work, which is a lockdown unit for Alzheimer's residents.

Staff and visitors can get into the unit, but we had to key in a code number to get out of the unit. An alarm would go off if any resident would happen to open one of the doors that led the street or the alley. There was also a camera that monitored those doors, which I did not know. My co-workers had explained to me that some of the residents liked to go to the back door, which led to the alley, because they were trying to go home. They also warned me to make sure that the residents I was responsible for had all been accounted for when the alarm went off. We also had to get to the back door to see if any one of the residents was successful in getting outside.

The alarm went off one day. I was checking to see if all of my assigned residents were accounted for, but I saw that the back door was opened. The resident who had opened the door was stopped and assisted back to his room. It took two CNAs to take him back, but I had no knowledge of what had happened. When I got to the door, I assumed that the resident had walked out, as I was not yet familiar with all the faces of the residents on our unit.

When I got outside, I saw a gentleman taking a walk behind our building. He looked exactly like one of the residents inside of the building. I told the old guy to come inside with me. I gently held onto his arm and tried to assist him inside. The man resisted and began to push away from me, while beating me on my arms, head, and shoulder with his wooden cane. I began to call my co-workers when one of them came outside. They told me that all of our residents were accounted for, and that the old man I was trying to get inside was not one of ours; he was a resident of the community.

I was truly embarrassed and annoyed with myself for trying to get the old man to go inside of the facility against his will, when all he wanted to do was take a walk before he ran into me.

After that day, Donna Gilroy, our charge nurse and team leader, made sure that everyone took turns making rounds all over the unit every thirty minutes, checking doors and looking for residents who may want to go out.

The residents who lived there were indeed allowed to go outside. They had a courtyard, and a beautiful area where they could sit outside and visit with their loved ones. But the doors that lead to the street or alley were off limits. Donna knew that working on a unit of Alzheimer's residents could be overwhelming sometimes. She let me know that she understood my frustrations and the problems with my assigned section of the unit. The residents there had Alzheimer's disease in every stage. It was interesting to see how they reacted in each stage of Alzheimer's while the disease was altering their lives.

Whenever we took a break together, we made sure we were away from the resident's family and visitors. Donna and I would talk about the residents. We had both been in the medical field over thirty years Even though Donna worked as a LPN and I was a CNA, we had still seen a lot. Although I had never worked on a unit with Alzheimer's sufferers in all stages at one time, we still agreed that these Alzheimer's sufferers are misunderstood, and having Alzheimer's does not mean that the person is crazy.

We also agreed that if we put ourselves in their place, and our family took us some place and left us there with people telling us what to do, and with people around us talking and acting strange, and we couldn't get out of there, we would question our own sanity, as well. Maybe not right away, but it wouldn't take long and that could be very frightening.

Some of the residents think that their parents are still alive, or that they have to go to work in the morning should not be persuaded otherwise, and we were trained not to argue with them. Insisting on something else will only confuse or upset them. It won't change their perception. The best thing to do is to be respectful and listen to them; they will eventually come back to their own reality.

Talking with Donna, sharing information, and working on the unit was a great help. Donna's talks helped me through a lot of emotional stress I endured while taking care of Mama.

I was glad I was transferred to the Valencia Villa Alzheimer's unit from the North Unit a long –trem Care Unit at Sunview Care Center.

I was a little reserved because even in orientation I'd heard about two CNAs who worked on that unit, who were very mean. They ran every CNA off who was sent to that unit to work. I also observed that they were both good CNAs. They were two very good workers; the residents were in very good hands with them. But I could plainly see that there really was a clique there, and I didn't want any part of it. Both of them were going to school at the time.

One was going to school to be a nurse, and the other one to be a cop. I was working a Baylor shift, and it was the first time I'd ever worked Baylor shift ,We work sixteen hour on Saturday and Sunday. When the Baylor shift is over on

Sunday night we were given credit for forty hours. The CNAs that worked from Monday through Friday never worked the weekend shift. I worked the entire weekend with them with no problems. The next weekend, I was transferred to another unit, the Alzheimer's Unit. I didn't like the Alzheimer's unit at first, but I was later grateful that I was transferred.

I met my friend Donna on the unit. Besides working great together with the residents, she and I hit it off the very first day we met. I could tell that Donna was from the old school like me, just by the way she interacted with the residents during the day.

Donna had one daughter and one grandchild. I told her about my four kids and five grandchildren. At the time, one of my daughters were expecting. We pulled out pictures to show off our grandkids. Donna's granddaughter was beautiful; her parents were interracial, and so was one of my granddaughter's parents. We both laughed and talked about how beautiful they were, and how much we loved them.

A few months after I'd worked on Valencia unit, two new CNAs who were friends of Donna's came to work with us at SunView Care Center: Carol Merhoffer and Tina Abrams. Carol was about five foot six, and she was a little heavy around the middle. She wore glasses, and had light brown hair. Carol was the type of co-worker who would take care of a resident even if the resident wasn't assigned to her for that day.

Carol was strong and gave the impression that she had the endurance of a Viking. Whenever Carol set her mind to do something, she got it done, no matter what she had to do to get it done.

Tina, on the other hand, was very timid. She was very heavy, and was about five foot five with brown hair and beautifully tanned skin. Tina had a very bad childhood, a bad marriage, and everyone took advantage of Tina's kindness. I always hoped that things would turn around for her. Tina was a team worker who was always there to help.

When I left SunView Care Center, Tina and Carol were still working there. They both had lost a lot of weight, and Tina was finally happy because she'd found someone to love her, and whom she loved very much. I hope it lasts forever. I'll never forget Carol or Tina. Whenever I was really depressed after I'd return from Florida visiting Mama, Carol or Tina was always there to offer a kind word, or to help me finish whatever I was doing.

Before that year was over, I got a call that let me know that I had to go back to Florida. I put in a request for the time off and got an approval from my D.O.N. and the super over my unit. Kim and Rhonda were very understanding about letting me have the time off. If ever there was an award to be given for "The Most Understanding Supervisor of the Year," I'd vote for them both every time.

I left the next week for Miami. When I got home, Mama looked worse. I couldn't believe how she'd changed from the last time that I'd seen her and Dad. The signs were there the last time I'd visited them, but I didn't want to believe that it could happen to my parents. Daddy was insisting that Mama would be all right and that he could handle everything. Sometimes it's hard to make the decision of what to do, when the other spouse is still alive and mentally functioning well. I knew that it was only a matter of time before Mama would need continuous care, and I'd have to move back to Miami.

We took Mama to see a neurologist again, Dr. Fischer, who prescribed medication that would slow down her memory loss, and he suggest a medication that may (or may not) increase Mama's appetite. When Daddy wheeled Mama out of the office in her wheelchair, I told the doctor that Mama had been crying a lot, but he said that the crying may not be a part of the dementia but a reaction to it. He said that Mama was grieving at the loss of her regular life, at the loss of control of her bodily functions, mental functions, and memory loss. It was final, I thought: I knew I had to come back to take care of Mama.

While visiting them, I noticed that Mama liked to sit in her recliner every day, while watching TV. Her legs, feet, and ankles were so swollen they didn't even look real. She had been sitting with her legs in the down position. The blood was not circulating properly. I positioned the recliner for Mama, keeping the bottom portion of her chair elevated for a few days and her legs went down. I wished that I could have stayed longer but I had to get back. Before I flew back, I told my sister Clara to keep a close watch on Mama and what to do to help her circulation. On my plane ride back to Phoenix, I kept thinking about Mama; it seemed like everything had changed overnight.

When I was a kid, and I needed Mama, she was always there to take care of me, and now I had a chance to do the same for her, and here I was leaving her again. Before Mama got sick, she was always there to make sure that everyone and everything was okay. She made sure that we all stuck together, and did the right thing, and now, Mama hardly know who's who.

When I got back to Phoenix, I got my business in order. Sometimes, I'd call back home to see how everything was coming along. When I did, Mama didn't answer the phone anymore, but that was okay because she'd stop making sense on the phone a long time before that. It seemed that the Alzheimer's disease was undoing everything in Mama's brain.

When I talked to Daddy on the phone, he said that something was wrong with Mama. He said that the medicine to increase Mama's appetite was not working. She wasn't eating and was losing a lot of weight. Daddy's voice sound shaky and worried and I wished I was there to comfort him.

I got another call from Miami the next day; it was Karen and Clara, who said that they were taking turns spending the night watching Mama, just in case she got up through the night and got into trouble while Daddy was sleeping. She had to be watched all the time. Daddy needed help, and they couldn't continue to spend the night very much longer.

I decided to help out for a while; Clara and Karen had families who needed them too. I knew that I had to fly back home to stay for a while. I prayed that Clara and Karen could hold on a little longer.

I went into a depression, and I cried a lot at work. I thought about Mama all the time, it seemed like I always had to take care of a resident who reminded me of Mama in some way. I knew that I had to go home soon.

CHAPTER ELEVEN

APRIL 2001

My sisters said that I should come home as soon as possible. I went back to Florida not knowing how long I'd be there. I'd already planned to go back but I had to change my plans even though I still had a lot of unfinished business to take care of. When I got off of the plane, I took a taxi to the house. When I got out of the taxi, Daveon, the neighborhood drunk, ran up to the taxi's door, and took my bag to our front door while I paid the taxi driver.

I knew that Daveon was only looking for a handout to quench his drug and alcohol addiction. When I got to the door, I was looking in my purse for my keys, and just as I'd expected, he wanted to "borrow" two dollars. It's always two dollars. And I thought, why does Daveon always want to borrow two dollars when he don't even have a job? But I turned around to answer Daveon; I could see that his skinny brown face had black and blue marks all over it, he had two black eyes, and two of his six front teeth had been knocked out.

"My goodness, what happened to you?" I asked, but before he could answer my question, Daddy came to the door and answered it for him.

"Go ahead and tell her how those guys kicked your butt for being stupid," Daddy blurted out.

Daveon followed me inside and put my bag down near the door, keeping his head down so his bruises wouldn't show.

"Why and where did this happened?" I asked Daveon.

From the look on Daddy's face, I could plainly see that he wanted to be the one to tell what happened, so I asked him.

"Go ahead, Dad, tell me what happened."

"He broke into some lady's house one night and her two sons had come back home, but Daveon didn't know that they were back." Daddy laughed and continued, "They watched him as he took her screen out of the window, and then they let him crawl inside…" Daddy laughed again. "When Daveon turned around, both of the guys beat the hell out of him."

Daveon was so annoyed, he didn't even stay around to see if he was going to get the two dollars he'd begged for.

Daddy said that maybe the bad experience Daveon had would change his way of life. But I didn't think so. It's going to take more than that to change him. I was more concerned about him and Mama living in that area. You can never tell what crack heads will do. I asked Daddy how he knew so much about Daveon's business.

Daddy said that he wanted Daveon to cut the grass for him, but he had not seen Daveon for a few days. He went to their house to see where he was, and his sister came to the door and told Daddy what had happened. Daveon's sister is a cop, so when the police were called that night, she'd come with another officer. Once they got inside, and she saw Daveon and realized that he was the burglar, she read him his rights and took him to jail as if he was a stranger.

The neighborhood had changed so much since I grew up there. I wondered if it was safe for them to live there anymore; a different breed of people had moved in.

It had been at least six months since I had seen either of them. When I walked into the living room, Mama was sitting in her chair. I leaned over and gave her a big hug and a kiss.

"Hey Mama, how are you?"

Mama started to laugh, she told me to turn around, and I did.

"Girl! You're just as fat as a butterball!" she said.

"Thank you, Mama," I said, and then I thought to myself, "Now, that's just what I needed to hear." I had put on at least ten pounds since I'd stopped smoking, and another ten since I'd moved to Arizona, so I didn't see the humor in the butterball jokes.

But I was concerned that she and Daddy both had lost so much weight, and Mama's memory was getting worse. She went into the bathroom to do her business. While I was talking to Daddy, she turned on the water and left it running. After hearing the water running for a while, I went in to see what had happened, but Mama was not in the bathroom; she was standing up in my old room (which is right next to the bathroom). She was looking around as if she was lost.

"Mama, are you all right?" I asked her.

"Get out of here! Leave me alone! I'm looking for my car keys!" she yelled out.

"Come on, Mama, let's go back into the living room," I said.

Daddy got up and came into the room, not looking very pleased.

"Come on, Amanda, cut that mess out. You know you don't have no car keys; you don't drive anymore," Daddy reminded her.

"Yes, I do! I just drove to the store with them," Mama insisted.

I told Daddy to calm down and to let her look for her keys until she gets tired. Mama looked in every drawer in her room for the car keys she never had but thought she'd lost. Mama talked to herself and looked for her keys for almost an hour, then finally she settled down and got into her recliner and went to sleep.

I cleaned the kitchen and made dinner. We ate, watched TV, and went to bed. After seeing how short-tempered Daddy was, I was glad I was there.

(SIX MONTHS LATER)

It was September already; I had been home six months and I wondered if I still had a job when I got back. I had taken a leave of absence, but I didn't realize that I'd be gone that long.

I prepared breakfast one morning, and made some phone calls. As I sat on the couch talking to a friend, I watched the morning news on TV. And as I watched, I could see the top of one of the Twin Towers smoking and in flames. I hung up the phone and turned the TV volume up; I was in shock. I couldn't believe my eyes. I saw a plane fly into the top of another building. I later learned that it was the Twin Towers that the plane had flown into. Then another news flash: The Pentagon had been attacked. Then another news flash: These plane crashes were terrorist attacks on the United States. And I thought to myself, "It's the end of the world!" I kept thinking about it and began to cry.

I felt scared. My heart felt shaky. Was the world coming to an end? I kept flipping the channels, but all I could see was the top of the Twin Towers smoking on every channel. I went to the front door to see what was happening outside. It's strange how we always think that we'll have our life in order by the time the world ended (or, at least I did). When in reality, the time is never right for life's interruptions.

On 9/11, I had a rude awaking: I'd already had an encounter with GOD when I was in Charlotte, but I had not fully submitted my life to him. This was certainly the time to receive Jesus as my Lord and Savior. Although I later learned the prayer to receive Jesus as my Lord and Savior, on that morning of 9/11, I didn't even know what to pray. I just prayed for forgiveness. I prayed for the people who were trapped in those buildings. I prayed for the families who lost their loved ones; and I prayed for the people who were on those planes.

I changed my lifestyle, and it was a change I struggled with for a while. I'd given my life to Jesus Christ. "Maybe now everything will get better for me," I thought. But It seemed like everything started getting worse.

I didn't know what was going to happen next. My world as I knew it was being turned upside down.

I'd asked GOD to help me understand why everything was going wrong. I was trying to do the right thing but things weren't getting any better. No matter what, I wasn't going back to the way I was before. I wished I'd listened to Mama when she was raising us. She tried to share her wisdom with us about God and about the Bible, but I wasn't listening then, and now, it was up to me to find my own way.

I had to get back to Phoenix, to prepare myself to come back home to take care of Mama until the end. I had an obligation to my job and other commitments still waiting for me in Arizona. Clara and Karen would have to take care of things until I got back home.

When I got back to Arizona, I went back to work. My position on Valencia Villa had been filled, and I was rehired to another unit. I went to the Central Unit to work this time. It was a unit for hospice patients and skilled nursing. I worked with a nurse who was very pleasant to work with; she was the LPN and team leader over that unit for the weekend.

She was a tall, skinny blonde who gave very good nursing care. Jude and I got along so well because we really cared about our residents, they were not just another room number to us. I remember one morning, not long after I'd started working on Central, I met an old gentleman who had been admitted the day before. He did not speak English or Spanish.

His family had brought him there for a period of rehab. The old gentleman was overwhelmed with the changes that had been made. People were talking to him and he did not understand what they were saying to him. Mr. Geno was eighty-nine years old and was not able to walk, but he was very strong.

Everyone who went into Mr. Geno's room would run out after being assaulted by him. I later learned that the other caregivers were trying to get Mr. Geno to do something, when he didn't understand what they were saying, and they also approached him with the wrong body language. Jude and I went into Mr. Geno's room together; we wanted him to take off his clothes and put on a hospital gown. Jude needed to examine him and I needed to bathe him.

When Mr. Geno began to shout at us in an unknown language, Jude realized that he was speaking Italian by some of the words he was shouting at us. Jude did not know how to speak Italian, but her husband and his family were Italian. Jude called her mother-in-law on the cordless phone and told her what problem we were having with Mr. Geno.

When Jude's mother-in-law agreed to talk to Mr. Geno, she gave him the phone with a very pleasant smile. He took the phone and talked to her mother-in-law. When he finished talking, he gave Jude the phone. His face looked more relaxed and he was smiling.

Jude learned from her mother–in-law that Mr. Geno agreed to cooperate with us, but he needed help to go to the bathroom. Mr. Geno had to make a B.M., and he didn't want to soil his clothes or the bed. We helped Mr. Geno get onto the bedside commode first, then we undressed him, Jude examined him, and I gave him a bath.

Mr. Geno's family never visited him. We often looked for someone to come in to comfort and console him. They all knew that he did not speak English, and was in a strange place where he couldn't communicate with anyone. Mr. Geno's family should have realized that he would be overwhelmed by the new surroundings and people who didn't speak Italian. But no one bothered to come and comfort Mr. Geno.

****

Many family members do not visit because they feel guilty for putting their loved ones in a home, and some are not sure that they are needed. I've talked to family members of residents and they've informed me that they knew that their mom or dad was angry with them, because they had put into a home. And they didn't know how to handle the anger, so they didn't visit.

****

Jude was a great nurse; I'll never forget working with her. Before I left SunView, Jude was going to school to be a registered nurse. I know that she will do well and be a very good RN.

When I wasn't working at SunView Care Center, I had a few private duty jobs. I took care of elderly ladies who needed help with their meals, a ride to the doctor's office, hair appointments, or just someone to talk to. I only stayed four or five hours a day with each of them.

One of my clients was Pauline Spears. Mrs. Spears and I became very good friends. She was a very nice lady, and was sometimes very funny. I'll always remember the good times I had while I was taking care of her. Mrs. Spears also had a daughter, Anita; we became good friends also. Anita introduced me to a club that she was a member of, the "Sisters of the Valley."

When I went to the meeting for the first time, I was very impressed. These were black women of all ages who had moved to Arizona from all over the country, were of different vocations and backgrounds, and had come together to have fun, share ideas, and bond with each other. I had not lived in Arizona that long, and although we were all women, it was the first time I'd seen that many blacks in one place at the same time since I had moved to the valley.

When I first moved to Arizona, I saw blacks sparingly. I was beginning to think that my daughter's family and I were the only other blacks living in the valley. During a conversation with Anita one day, I told her of my new experience in becoming a believer. I told her that I needed guidance. I needed someone to show me how to be a good Christian. I didn't know what I should do next.

I'd watched the Christian channel, but I needed more. Anita invited me to her church, the Antioch Church of God in Christ. When I visited her church for the first time, it made me want to know more. The order of the church service was different from the Catholic church service. I was a born Catholic, but had strayed away and stopped going for years. But the message was one I needed to hear. The pastor's message convinced me that GOD really did love me, and that he knew me. The pastor's entire message was like fuel in my tank, because I was giving out and was about to give up. I was hungry for every word the pastor delivered that morning. I continued to visit Antioch and it was a great help. The last time I visited Antioch was in 2003. I'd be leaving the next week to go back to Miami to take care of Mama.

Pastor Logan preached a message that Sunday about getting rid of negative people around you. It seemed as if he was talking directly to me. I felt uneasy in my seat, I kept thinking, "He couldn't possibly know what happened when I was home last year." That sermon seemed to be designed just for me. It seemed everything the pastor said was what I needed to hear. The only thing missing in the sermon was my name. There were people who I needed to cut out of my life when I went back to Miami. I knew that when I returned to Miami, my faith would be tested again, and I'd need that Armor of GOD that the pastor was talking about.

As days passed, I prepared myself to go back to Miami. I thought about my friends, and some of my family members, and how they would receive me when I let them know that there would be no compromising. I knew I had to move on and stop trying to hold onto negative relationships.

I got the phone call I'd been expecting for months, I needed to go home to take care of Mama. My sisters sent me a one-way ticket to return to Miami. I dropped everything that I was doing and flew back home.

Clara picked me up from the airport. She told me that Mama had lost an awful lot of weight, and that Daddy had also lost quite a bit of weight. I kept trying to imagine how they'd look with the weight lost this time; the last I visited, I tried to put some of the weight back on them. The images of how they were going to look, kept showing up in my mind.

When I walked into the house, Mama was sitting in her recliner watching TV. Daddy was sitting in his recliner watching Mama watch TV. He was nervously shaking his feet and rubbing his shiny head. I sat down on the couch so that I could get a good look at both of them. I looked into both of their small, frail faces, and I made myself hold back my tears.

When I realized how much weight both of them had lost, it just broke my heart. It seemed as though Mama had lost at least sixty pounds. She'd lost so much weight her dentures looked too big for her face. Her high cheekbones seemed to set out more, and her face seemed to have sunk in. When I looked into her eyes, the Mama I knew wasn't in there.

Daddy had lost at least thirty pounds. His once-thick and healthy body had melted into that of a thin and frail old man. Both of their features had changed; they almost looked like strangers to me. I wanted to scream when I saw Daddy stand. He walked over to kiss Mama on the forehead, and his belt could almost go around his waist twice.

Mama seemed to have been having a good day. I talked to them for a while, and then I excused myself and I went to the bathroom. When I got into the bathroom, I sat on the edge of the bathtub and I cried until I had no more tears. I had to get myself together so that I could go back out into the living room. I didn't want them to know how upset I was. I did everything I could think of to keep from looking at Mama, because I wanted to cry every time I looked in her direction. I wanted to hold Mama and tell her that everything was going to be all right, and even if I couldn't make it all right, I'd go to the limit trying to.

When I looked into Mama's eyes, I could see that some of her personality was gone. I cried because the Mama I'd known since I was a kid wasn't there anymore, and I wished that I could have her back.

When I came back home to take care of Mama, I began to keep a journal, and I tried to make entries in it every day but I couldn't. You see, there were days when my heart was too heavy to even think about writing what had happened that day.

Some days, Mama was sad and she cried because she didn't know why she'd forget things, or why she couldn't concentrate long enough to prepare a meal, or even remember simple things like my name.

Sometimes, Mama would have a flash of sanity, and she'd ask, "What's happening to me?" I could see that Mama couldn't explain what she was feeling. Her mind seemed to be in a fog.

Some days, Mama was happy; she'd remember things that had happened a long time ago. But somehow, she couldn't remember what we had done or where we had been the day before.

CHAPTER TWELVE

ENTRIES OF MY JOURNAL

The remaining pages of this book are entries I made while I was taking care of Mama every day. Some days, I was not strong enough to write anything, while other days I could write detailed entries.

As I write this book, I am fighting back my tears as I share with you another story of how the Alzheimer's disease can affect the family life of its victims.

For those of you who are courageous enough to be the caregiver for your parent (or parents): Please know that once you trust GOD, love and understanding will get you through the rest. It will equip you with the strength to meet the tasks that lie ahead of you.

****

May 20, 2004

Today, Mama had company. It was someone she and Daddy had known from the old neighborhood, but Mama had no idea of who he was; she couldn't even remember his face or his name. But she greeted him with open arms and welcomed him into her home as if it was her very first time meeting him. The friend who was visiting her understood what was going on with Mama, and acted accordingly.

* * * *   * * **

****

May 25, 2004

After dinner tonight, I sat in the chair next to Mama and we watched TV together. Dad had said good night and went to bed. Mama and I laughed and talked about the movie. I wasn't sure if Mama understood the movie (or why we were laughing) but she seemed to be enjoying herself. Mama got very quiet and sad. I asked Mama what was the matter, and she answered,

"Where is Mama?" Her mind had wondered away again.

"Mama, your mother is dead," I answered. I didn't want to be so blunt, but I wanted to keep her as close to reality as possible

Mama put both of her hands on top of her head, then she looked at me. She said that if she had been going back home to Tallahassee every year like she should have, then she would have known that her mother was dead.

"When did Mama die?" she asked me with a face full of tears.

"Mama, your mom has been dead for over forty years," I answered. Seeing Mama reliving her mother's death made me cry too.

I suffered with Mama whenever she had a flashback or a memory lapse. I was caught up in the moment with her because Mama cried like she'd heard that her mother was dead for the first time. I was glad that she accepted my answer about her mom's death, and not argue or tell me that I had lied, like she'd done in other situations.

I cried for Mama's confusion, and I cried because Mama had realized that parts of her life and memory was missing. She couldn't put the pieces together, and she didn't know why.
****

Sometimes, trying to convince the Alzheimer's sufferer that their parents are not alive or insisting on something else, may confuse them more at that moment, because they are in a different place and time.
****

**************   ************

May 28, 2004

I had a long talk with Daddy tonight, because sometimes, he thinks that if he talks tough or if he fusses at Mama, she'll just snap out of her confusion.

Daddy's frustration keeps Mama upset too. When Mama's having a bad day and she's confused, Daddy gets upset with her, and when Mama feels his hostility toward her, she cries because she don't know why he's upset with her.

When I saw how dad reacts to Mama, I'm glad that I came home to take care of Mama, so that she wouldn't be subjected to the mental abuse from Daddy. I know his verbal abuse is unintentional, but Mama still needs to be protected from that kind of behavior; she doesn't know what she's doing.

I also understand that Dad's still trying to hold onto the wife that he used to know, but she's gone now. And no matter how tough he talks to her, it wont reverse what has already happened to Mama.

**************   ****************

May 30, 2004

This morning at breakfast, I put Mama's breakfast plate down in front of her just like any other morning. Daddy blessed the food, and asked Mama how she felt. Mama just looked at him she never answered him; it was as though Mama was in another world.

Then Mama looked at her breakfast plate as if she didn't know what to do with it. I told Mama that the food wasn't hot, and that she could go ahead and eat, but Mama picked up the cup of coffee I'd made for her and poured it into her breakfast plate and all over the table.

Daddy got upset, but I told him that it was okay. She was having a bad day. Mama began to cry out loud but I began to cry inside. I knew that Mama was getting worse and that there was nothing I could do to stop the progress of that terrible disease.

*********** ************

June 5, 2004

I went into the room this morning to get Mama washed and dressed for the day, but she was having a severe pain in her left leg and in her left hip. Every time I tried to help Mama get out of bed, she'd screamed with pain.

I let her stay in bed a little longer, at least until she felt better (after I gave her something to help ease her pain). Mama was able to move better but she was even more confused. I knew that it was going to be one of those days but I got her up anyway.

************ **********

June 8, 2004

Today, Mama had another bad day. She refused to eat breakfast or lunch. And by the time I served dinner, she'd had two fainting spells. Mama's also a diabetic.

I've made an appointment with Dr. Sanchez; we'll take her to the HMO clinic tomorrow.

************** ***********

June 9, 2004

Today, we took Mama to see Dr. Sanchez, and he said that we were going to need help from hospice and that Mama was going downhill very quickly.

He said that the most important thing for us to do now is to keep Mama comfortable, pain-free, and satisfied as much as possible.

Dr. Sanchez said that he was going to put in an order to have someone from VITAS (the hospice organization) come out to visit Mama at home. When Dr. Sanchez said that Mama needed to be on hospice, I knew that Mama was in bad shape.

When we got back home, I called my sisters and had them come over to the house. I told my sisters and Daddy what the doctor had said about putting Mama on hospice. But they still didn't understand that if Mama needed to be on hospice, that she was getting worse. I told them that VITAS would be helping me take care of Mama, and that Mama was getting a little weaker. They were crying and were very upset.

After seeing their bad reaction to that news about Mama getting weaker, I knew I couldn't tell them that Dr. Sanchez also said that Mama only had six months to live. I knew I had to keep it to myself for a while.

I knew Mama's fate was going to have to be a personal journey for me, and I'd have to carry it alone to keep our family from falling apart too soon. If I would have told them everything that Dr. Sanchez had said, it would have been impossible for me to take care of Mama properly, with all of them mourning her death before she'd even died.

It would have only been more confusing for Mama.

She needed all of the positive energy and support that was available.

************** ************

June 10, 2004

Today, Mama has been rather hostile. This morning, she didn't want me to help her out of bed, wash her, or even touch her, so I let her sleep in a little later.

When I went back, Mama still wanted to fight. She'd wet her diaper and didn't want to be changed. Mama didn't want to cooperate with anything I tried to do for her today. I have to pray about this.

I love her, and I know she doesn't know what she's doing.

*********************   ***************

June 15, 2004

Today the nurse from VITAS said that she thinks that Mama should see the doctor about her leg again. She's sending Mama to North Shore Hospital, to find out why Mama is experiencing so much pain.

******************   ******************

June 20, 2004

Today, Mama came home from the hospital. Her appetite is very poor, and she can't stand up on her walker anymore. She seemed to have lost a lot of ground since she was admitted into the hospital. At least, she was walking around on her walker before she was admitted. We expected Mama to be stronger and do better when she came home. I believe that if I had not come home to take care of Mama, she would not have lasted two months.

Whenever I help Mama out of the bed I have to put her into a wheelchair now.

Mama is wheelchair-bound now; it's the only way I can move her around the house.

************************ ********************

June 25, 2004

Today, I realized that Mama's condition is affecting Daddy in a negative way. I hope that Mama's condition does not send him into a depression, because he cries when I bring Mama to the table in the morning to have breakfast.

Daddy says that he can't stand to see Mama being pushed around in the wheelchair. Daddy yells at Mama to make her stand up on her walker. Daddy refuses to believe that Mama can't walk anymore. The walker is a thing of the past now.

Whenever I get Mama out of bed, I have to lift her from the bed to the wheelchair. Sometimes, Daddy shouts at Mama, telling her to stand up, and she'd look into his angry face and began to cry.

Daddy's denial of Mama's condition keeps him frustrated, which leads to the verbal abuse.

******************* **********

June 28, 2004

After we had dinner tonight, I got Mama washed up and ready for bed. As I was taking Mama into the bedroom that she and Daddy still share, I pulled back the cover on Mama's side of their king-sized bed. I could see that she couldn't bring herself to get into the bed with (who she thought at that moment to be) a stranger.

Mama said that I had taken her to the wrong room, because there was someone already in the bed and she didn't know who he was. I realized that she was no doubt scared and confused at that moment. Mama held my hand as tight as I would have held her hand when I was frightened as a child.

I didn't push the issue; I took Mama into the guest room and talked to her until her mind was somewhat clear again. When I took Mama back into her room, Daddy was gone. He was in the living room watching TV.

Once I got Mama into the bed, she wanted to know where Dad was. She wouldn't go to sleep until she saw him lying next to her. I pleaded with Daddy to go back in the room with Mama. Although Daddy was very angry, he did what I'd asked him to do.

******************* **********

June 30, 2004

Today, Daddy's doctor's office called. They want Daddy to come in next week for his prostate surgery. Daddy has a super-pubic in-dwelling catheter in his stomach. They wanted to try reconstructive surgery so he'll be able to urinate from his penis.

I pray that the surgery is successful, because I don't know what I'd do if his health starts to fail too.

****************** *************

CHAPTER THIRTEEN

July 4, 2004

I talked to Clara and Karen last night and I told them not to worry about trying to share the holiday(July 4th) with us, because Mama don't know what day it is, and Daddy's too angry to enjoy it. I told them to go ahead and enjoy the holiday with their families.

I wanted to make some burgers and put just a few ribs in the oven for the three of us, but Daddy insisted that it was a waste of time and money.

He seems to be angry all of the time. Nothing is ever right. We fuss a lot now. I let Daddy have his way when he wants to fight with me. I just don't want him to upset Mama.

************** ************

July 10, 2004
Mama is in bed most of the time now. I try to get her out of bed at least twice a day to eat her meals. She still has good days and bad days. On Mama's good days, she still has flashbacks of things that happened years ago.
********************* ****************

July 15, 2004
Daddy came home from the hospital today. His surgery was unsuccessful and he is very unhappy. Dad is sleeping in the guest room now. The hospital sent him home with two catheters, and he's still draining from his incision and it may be infectious. He'll do better in a room by himself. I wouldn't want Mama to catch anything.

Ellen Abel

Dad is even angrier now than he was before he had the surgery, but I guess he has every reason to be.

***************   **********

July 17, 2004

Mama has noticed that Dad's been in bed all day. When I tell her what has happened with Dad, she'll forget and ask why he's in bed ten minutes later. It's driving me crazy.

Mama cries because Daddy's not sleeping in the bed with her anymore. She calls for Daddy all night and it's beginning to wear on my nerves.

Mama wants Dad to get into the bed with her. Daddy sounds very angry and hostile when he shouts from the guest room that he's sick infected and needs to sleep alone.

Daddy is angry about his condition, and he's angry because Mama is sick. He's feeling lonely because his wife and his best friend has disappeared right before his eyes.

Sometimes, when Daddy's having a bad day, his behavior is very nasty toward me. But it's okay. I understand what he's going through.

****************   ***********

July 23, 2004

Today, Mama seems to be weak. I tried to put her on the bedside commode this morning but she's not bearing any weight at all on either of her legs.

It's getting harder to get Mama out of bed. I'll only get Mama up for one meal a day now. I hope that I could hold out.

*********************   ************

July 27, 2004

Today when the VITAS nurse came, she said that I should leave Mama in bed. Since Mama can't stand up at all, it would be unsafe for both of us to try and get her in and out of bed.

************   **********

July 29, 2004

Today, Mama's in good spirits, even though she's not able to get out of bed. She asked me if I'd stay in the room to talk with her, and nothing I know could have pleased me more than that. Whenever Mama is in good spirits, she still seems to only remember things that happened long ago. Mama was telling me how she hated to send her little girls away, when they were small, then she started to cry again.

I realized that she'd gone back to another place in time. Mama was having a flashback about the time she had a nervous breakdown.

Her mother was making a surprise visit to Miami to see her. She took a taxi from the Greyhound Bus station to bring her to our house. The taxi driver had been drinking. He went to sleep while driving and ran off of a bridge, and they both drowned. Once Mama got the news about her mother's drowning, it overwhelmed her, and Mama had a nervous breakdown.

Mama sent my sisters and me back to her hometown of Tallahassee, Florida.

Bobbie and I lived with Grandma Rosa Lee and Grandpa Sanford for a year.

Annette lived with Mama's brother, and Clara lived with Daddy's sister. (Karen wasn't born yet.)

Grandpa Sanford was blind, and he liked to walk around the neighborhood. Grandpa Sanford knew the neighborhood so well, he could almost take a walk by himself.

I was about five years old. Bobbie was in the first grade.

I stayed home with Grandma and my job was to take Grandpa Sanford for a walk after lunch every day. I guess I was his seeing eye dog. Anyway, we went for a walk one day, and we had walked the same way we always walked every day. On the way back, we had to walk down a hill and walk into an area where there was a ditch on each side of the path. But

Grandpa Sanford decided that we were going the wrong way. He wanted to turn around and go back, and the way he wanted to go was into a ditch.

I kept telling him that he was going the wrong way, but Grandpa Sanford said that I was lying. He took about two steps and tumbled into a ditch. When I looked down into the ditch, I began to laugh. Grandpa's hat and his white cane were laying on top of him, and his starched and ironed brown khaki pants and shirt had dead leaves and grass all over. I'd tried to tell him that he was walking into a hole but he just wouldn't listen, and now he looked as if he'd been playing in the ditch.

I got down into the ditch to try to help Grandpa Sanford, but he wouldn't let me touch him. A man passing by had seen Grandpa when he'd fallen and hurried over to help Grandpa get out of the ditch. He made sure that Grandpa Sanford had no broken bones and was able to walk by himself.

Once he saw that Grandpa Sanford was okay, he got back into his car and drove off. On the way back home, I held Grandpa's hand as we walked up the hills and down the paths. On the way back home, Grandpa Sanford seemed a little confused but he walked in the direction I told him to.

Grandpa Sanford had always walked around the whole neighborhood with his white cane. I couldn't understand what had happened to Grandpa Sanford when he insisted on going the wrong way. (I think Grandpa Sanford had a little dementia that no one talked about.)

I couldn't wait to get Grandpa home, so Grandma could see how dirty he'd gotten by not listening to me. I kept thinking, "Oh boy, Grandpa! Grandma Rosa Lee is really going to be mad at you for getting so dirty."

"Grandma never liked it when your clothes got dirty," I thought. "And the way Grandpa looked, he was really going to get it," I kept thinking.

As mean as he'd been to me that day, I wanted Grandma to put his white stick all over his back, just like she would done if I'd gotten my clothes that dirty.

But boy, was I ever wrong about Grandma Rosa Lee. Grandpa Sanford told Grandma that he had fallen in a ditch and it was all my fault. I was punished for it anyway. I cried because it wasn't my fault, and I cried because Grandma didn't believe me.

When Bobbie came home from school that day, I told her what had happened to me. But Bobbie was still sad because she'd gotten punished for burning her school dress in the fireplace.

The weather was cold that morning, and the rooms in grandma's house were not heated that well. Bobbie went into the living room to put her dress in front of the fireplace to get it warm before she put it on. She'd seen our Aunt Richie do it dozens of times when she was getting ready for school. But Bobbie had put her dress too close to the fire that morning and she burned the end of it. Grandma said that Bobbie didn't like her school dress and that's why she burned it.

That evening, we decided that it was time for us to leave Grandma's house. We were going back to Miami where our mother was when we first moved with her. Every time we'd hear someone ask Grandma whose kids we were, she'd always say, "These are my son Robert's kids. He married Amanda and they live down in Miami with the bright lights, big city!"

Bobbie and I decided that we were going back home, and it would be easy to find Miami by its bright lights in the big city.

By the time we finished our dinner, we only had a few hours to go out to play before the sun went down. When Grandma sent us outside to play, we had no time to waste. We walked down a path that took us to the highway. After we got to the end of the path, we would have to cross a four-lane highway to get to the other side. As we looked across the frightening street, we could see the bright lights just beyond the trees on the other side.

"That's it!" we said to each other, "That's where Mama is."

"Ellen, look over there — can you see the bright lights?" Bobbie asked, as she held my hand even tighter to make an attempt to dash across the highway.

"Yeah! I see it" I answered. I still remember how shaky I felt. I just wanted to get home to Mama. I would have followed Bobbie anywhere, as long as she got me home safely.

Our only problem was figuring out how we were going to get across that highway safely. I had already seen how cats and dogs had been torn apart trying to get across, and I didn't want to join them.

The cars were racing down the highway as fast as we could bat our eyes. It seemed as though we'd never get across that highway, and I was losing hope. Hours had passed and we were still holding hands, waiting for a break to get across the highway.

But by that time, Grandma had sent everyone out looking for us. We could hear their voices calling for us in the distance.

"BOBBIE! ELLEN!"

When we heard their voices come closer, we got nervous and made an attempt to dash across the highway, but the car horns blew so loud, it scared us back to our waiting spot. Finally Mary (one of the big kids from the neighborhood) came walking up the path. She asked us if we needed help getting across the highway. She said that she needed to cross the highway too, and that she'd take us with her. We nodded our heads indicating that yes, we needed help. After Mary got our confidence, she told us that it would be easier to cross if we'd follow her down the path a little farther, and there, she'd show us how to get across.

Bobbie and I smiled at each other, happy that we were on our way home to see Mama. We held hands and hurried behind Mary, walking as fast as our little feet would carry us. But she had lied to us! She took us right into the hands of our enemy (Grandma), who was waiting for us with her paddle. We could see the rage in Grandma's eyes, and we knew what we were in for when Grandma got us back home. Grandma told us to walk in front of her, and every time we'd slow down, we'd get paddled. When we got home, we got our punishment and went to bed.

After that day, Grandma told everyone who would listen that I'd pushed Grandpa Sanford into a ditch, Bobbie tried to burn up her school clothes, and then we tried to run away. It seemed like we were going to relive that day forever. A year later, Daddy came back to get us. Mama looked and acted the way she had before she'd gotten sick.

We all went back to Miami to live, but every time we'd go back to Tallahassee to visit for the summer, Bobbie and I would stick to Mama like glue; we wouldn't let her out of our sight. We never wanted her to leave us behind in Tallahassee again.

*********** ************** *************

CHAPTER FOURTEEN

JOURNALING THE MIDDLE STAGES

August 3, 2004

I'm having a bad day today.

I cried all night. Every time I'd go in to turn Mama or to change her, I'd break down when I get back into my room. Seeing Mama in the state that she's in is killing me. I know that Mama was leaving me soon and there was no way that I could save her or make her better. I have to just take it. I don't know how long I can hang on like this.

When I was a little girl, sometimes Mama would get up with me during the night and take care of me. When she kissed me on the cheek, I'd feel better, and by the morning, I'd be all right. I kissed Mama on the cheek last night, and pretended that she'd be all right this morning.

****

August 8, 2004

Today, I took the twin beds out of the guest room. I turned that room into a hospital room for Mama. Now I can move around in it and take care of Mama without being cramped.

Daddy does not approve of Mama having a hospital bed. He says that I'm going too fast. Daddy says that I'm taking Mama to a point of no return, and she's not that bad. (Daddy's having a hard time accepting Mama's sickness. "First the wheelchair, and now a hospital bed?" he says.) Daddy's upset that Mama can't be the wife and mother we once knew, and I wish that Daddy would accept it. But he's still trying to hold on to yesterday, and those days are gone forever.

********************   ****************

August 10, 2004

Daddy eats his meals alone now. Mama is confined to her bed and she won't be joining him to eat meals anymore. I try to eat at least one meal with him to try to keep him from feeling so alone. Daddy has always been the type of person who liked to talk while he's eating his meals, but he hardly says a word to me these days.

Each morning, before Daddy goes in to eat breakfast, he stands in the doorway of Mama's room, and he just looks at her. Sometimes, when I'm in the room turning Mama onto her other side, I can feel Daddy watching from the doorway and when I look up at him, his eyes are full of tears. I want to cry too, but I know that I have to be strong for both of us. Yet my heart cries out, "GOD, PLEASE HELP US!"

*******   ****************   *************

August 12, 2004

Mama's appetite is very poor, and she is deteriorating quickly. I have to try and force fluids on Mama; she hardly drinks anything. Only GOD'S Grace is keeping me strong enough to watch Mama go through this; my heart breaks every time she refuses eat or take a drink when I offer it to her.

************   ************

August 15, 2004

Last night as I laid in bed, I accepted the fact that Mama is going to leave me, but knowing this and accepting it are very different. I've known for a while that Mama didn't have long to be with us, because Dr. Sanchez told me so. But last night, I accepted it in my heart. Although it's painful for me, I now have the strength to release Mama. I don't want her to suffer anymore. I want her to rest in peace.

***************   ***********

August 16, 2004

The VITAS nurse ordered oxygen for Mama today. Mama was having problems breathing last night. Daddy looks

Taking Care of Mama

very nervous; he gets up all during the night, because of the machine. He thinks that Mama may stop breathing.

I keep telling myself that Mama is going to leave me, but it won't be the end for her. It will be a glorious beginning for her in heaven.

I'm taking care of Mama the best way I know how in this life. But I want Mama to be on the right track when she leaves me. I want to help her rededicate her life to GOD.

So I asked Mama if she could hear me, and she said, "Yeah, baby, I hear you."

Then I asked her to repeat after me, and she said okay.

Then I said, "FATHER, I CONFESS THAT JESUS IS MY LORD."

Mama repeated it, and then I said, "I MAKE HIM LORD OF MY LIFE RIGHT NOW."

Then Mama said, "That's right, baby," and I told her to repeat it, and she did. So I continued to say:

"I BELIEVE IN MY HEART THAT YOU RAISED JESUS FROM THE DEAD."

When Mama repeated that, I told Mama to say, "THANK YOU FOR FORGIVING ME FOR ALL OF MY SINS."

Mama repeated everything, and then she said, "Thank you, baby. I'm glad that you're thinking about Jesus too."

I cried and I kissed Mama's face.

**************** ************* ************

August 17, 2004

Mama had a busy night last night; every time I went in to turn her on her other side, she had pulled the sheet and blanket off of herself. Even her gown was off; Mama was naked and had folded everything into a neat little pile lying right next to her. I asked Mama what she had been doing. She said that she was tired from doing the laundry. I knew Mama's arms had to be tired — she'd been lying on her back, folding a big blanket, sheet, and her gown in the dark.

********** ***********

103

August 18, 2004

Today, Mama started doing a new thing: She keeps her eyes closed all of the time. Even when Mama talks to you, her eyes are closed.

**********　********

August 20, 2004

Mama seems to have shut everyone out; she won't talk to us anymore.

I think that Mama is making a transition between this world and the supernatural world and she need this time to herself. It hurts me to know that Mama realizes that she's dying, and there is nothing that I can do to help.

******************　************

August 21, 2004

As much as I have tried to avoid it, Mama is still getting a bed sore on her butt. The nurse says that while Mama's not eating, her body has a protein deficiency. Her body is so low in protein that when the nurse pinched the skin together on Mama's arm, it stuck (a sign that her skin will be breaking down very quickly).

************　************

August 22, 2004

Mama cried and called for Daddy all night last night. Daddy almost pulled his catheter out when he jumped up to see what had happened to Mama. When he got to the door, he asked Mama, "What's wrong?" and she said that her brother was there visiting her.

"What brother? Where is he?" Daddy asked.

"It's Sonny Boy; don't you see him sitting there?" Mama answered as she pointed to the chair.

"Damn that chair! There's no one there!" Daddy shouted. He went into his room and slammed the door, but I could hear him crying in the late hours of the night.

**********   ************

August 23, 2004

The VITAS nurse said that Mama has a urinary tract infection. She said that Mama is not drinking enough water. I gave Mama a cool glass of water but she refused it. The nurse told me to try it again later. I did, but Mama only took a sip.

*************   **********

August 24, 2004

Nothing seems to please Daddy anymore; he's been as mean as hell. I asked him why he's so angry, and he began to tell me about the rotten childhood he'd had.

He was his mother's oldest child of six, but the stepson of a father who didn't even acknowledge him as one of his own. As I listened to him, I could see how after all of these years, Daddy's anger had festered into bitterness.

But I also realize that Daddy is angry now because he's losing the only person that he feels really loves him and has cared about him all of these years. Mama has been his wife, his lover, his friend, and his consultant for sixty-five years, and now she's going to leave him.

******************   **********

August 26, 2004

I went in to check on Mama last night, and she had a high fever — 103.2. The VITAS nurse had already left some medication for her in case she got a temp like that. When I checked Mama again, it had gone down to 99.0.

***************   **********

August 27, 2004

This morning, Mama's temp was 103.2 again. Her body was hot and she's fighting me whenever I touch her. It was hard, but I held Mama down long enough to insert another one of the suppositories in her, and put ice packs under her arms, her groin, and the back of her neck. Mama didn't like it and she let me know that she didn't. She called me every name that she could think of. I laughed and welcomed Mama's anger — because at least she was talking to me.

*************   ********

August 28, 2004

Today the RN, Ms. Elizabeth Davis (the nurse working on Mama's case) told me that she's ordering continual care for Mama. Someone from VITAS will come tonight to stay with Mama around the clock. That really took a lot of weight off of my shoulders. At least, I'll be able to sleep at night. I am really worried about the hurricanes; we are having them back-to-back.

I keep thinking what I would do if we were out of electricity for more than two or three days. I keep the TV on the news station, and whenever the hurricanes are reported heading in our direction, I keep the air conditioner as cold as we could stand it, so that if we are without electricity, the house would stay cool longer. I always keep Mama's hospital bed in the high position so that it would be easier for me to take care of her in case the electricity wasn't available for days.

The VITAS nurse finally came, and I was glad to see her. VITAS is the best thing that ever happened to hospice patients. I thank GOD for VITAS and I thank GOD for Liz who was the hospice nurse over Mama's case.

***************   ********

CHAPTER FIFTEEN

THE LAST STAGES

September 1, 2004

Mama's still not eating much; one small cup of applesauce is all she had today.

**************** ***********

September 3, 2004

Mama sleeps most of the day now and I stand by the bed trying to get her to eat something, or at least say something to me. When she refuses to eat or talk, I sit by her bed and read the scriptures, or write in my journal.

I need to advise Clara, Karen, and Daddy of Mama's situation, so that they can begin to release Mama in their hearts in their own way. Letting go is the hardest part, and I have to let them handle it as best they know how.

I have known that Mama was given six months to be with us, when the doctor put her on hospice in June. I've tried to keep things around this house as normal as possible, and since Daddy is here with her every day, I didn't want him to be sad and grieve for her so hard, but now he has to know. In the back of his mind, he may already know that Mama doesn't have that much time with him, but when you put it into words, it makes dealing with the situation that much more of a reality because it's final. Clara and Karen have jobs, and little ones to care for, and they're not around to see the day-to-day deterioration of Mama's mind and body, so they'll cry and be overwhelmed when I tell them that Mama will be leaving us soon.

That is also why I choose to keep Mama's illness to myself. It's been lonely and painful for me, but it was the best way to keep our family from falling apart while Mama has been going through her illness. Mama need all of our support, for as long as possible.

Tonight, I'll break the news to them. I'll tell Daddy sometime today.

************** ************** ***********

September 15, 2004

When I helped the nurse turn Mama onto her side this morning, she opened her eyes and looked at me. I offered her a drink, but she refused it. As I talked to Mama, I knew that she wasn't going to answer me. But she looked at me as though she was trying to tell me something. I took Mama's hand and asked her if she wanted to say something to me. I could see the tears coming from her eyes.

I kept saying to her, "Mama, what's wrong?"

She began to squeeze my hand very tightly. I knew that something was wrong so I called the nurse to come to the bed to see what was wrong with Mama. The nurse came to the bed and checked her. Mama closed her eyes. The tightness from her grip was relaxed, and her hand was now limp. I looked at the nurse but she said Mama would be all right.

I think that the nurse just wanted me to feel relaxed. She already knew that Mama was having a stroke. But in Mama's condition, there was nothing to do but keep her comfortable.

Two hours later, it was time to turn Mama again. I looked at Mama's face to see if she was awake yet, and the right side of her face was sagging down.

She didn't look like the same skinny, frail-faced person that I'd gotten used to looking at; her face had changed somehow. The nurse called someone on the phone to report Mama's condition. I stood by Mama's bedside, crying and holding her hand, then I called out to her, "Mama? Mama?" a few times, but there was no response.

I held up Mama's limp hands and kissed them, and placed them back at her side. I prayed that she didn't suffer, and then I cried softly so that Daddy couldn't hear me. I didn't want to upset him. How would I find the words to tell him that Mama had a stroke on top of everything else?

********* ************   ******* ******

September 29, 2004

It's been two weeks since Mama's stroke. Daddy doesn't say very much anymore.

When he gets up in the morning, before he does anything, he stands at Mama's room door and just looks at her. He never goes into the room. Sometimes he cries, and sometimes he just shakes his head and grunts.

As I watch him from afar, I cry inside and I pray that GOD will give Daddy peace, and help him to accept Mama's absence when she is gone from his sight.

Daddy will never be able to release Mama from his heart. They have been together so long, Mama is just like another limb on his body.

***************   *******************

CHAPTER SIXTEEN

DOES MAMA KNOW THAT
SHE'S DYING?

October 3, 2004

I called Mama's sister this morning (Aunt Cider). I wanted to let her know how poorly Mama was doing. She lives in the same area as Mama, and has lived there for the past thirty-five years. Mama is one of sixteen brothers and sisters, and all but three have passed away. The Hannah family was one of the biggest families within Leon County in Tallahassee, Florida, where they were all born. Some moved to different parts of the country, but most of them remained in Florida.

Aunt Cider moved to Miami when I was still in high school, but it seems like she's lived there forever. Aunt Cider's health is also very poor. She has a severe case of gout, only one kidney, and sight in only one eye. I've chosen not to tell any of Mama's brothers or sisters every detail of her sickness, because they have their own sickness and issues to deal with.

Mama only has one living brother, Caleb Hannah. He's blind and lives in Tallahassee. Mama also has a younger sister, Sarah, who lives in Tallahassee. She's had a double mastectomy and other health problems. Her oldest sister is still living, but she lives in a nursing home in Tampa, but she's been in a coma for almost a year now.

✶✶✶✶✶✶✶✶✶✶✶✶✶   ✶✶✶✶✶✶✶✶✶✶✶✶✶

October 5, 2004

Aunt Cider came over to see Mama today, and some of her children and grandchildren came along with her. But Mama's condition didn't let her recognize any of her family. Mama just stares into space. Many of our friends and family are visiting us since they've gotten the news that Mama's getting worse. It seems like every day has been full of tears and sadness lately.

*********************** ***********

October 10, 2004

Last night, Clara and I talked about giving Mama a birthday party before the day of her actual birthday, because she looks as if she's slipping farther and farther away from us each day.

Liz (the VITAS hospice nurse) came over to see Mama this morning. I told her of our plan about Mama's birthday and she agreed. It didn't look like Mama would be around until her birthday, which was on October 23.

Liz even talked to Daddy about Mama's condition today. Even though I'd already told him about Mama, Liz's confirmation made it a reality. He seemed to accept the fact that Mama was really dying, and that it was final. Daddy laid back in his recliner and closed his eyes. It seemed as though reality had finally sunk in. Mama was going to leave him; she would be gone from his sight forever; and then Daddy cried. I cried with him as I stood off in the kitchen.

My heart throbbed with grief.

That night, Daddy began to call all of the relatives to let them know what was going on with Mama. As Daddy made each phone call, I listened as he talked. Sometime he'd be strong and sometimes he'd break down and cry. A dagger went through my heart every time I saw my daddy cry.

**************** *****************

October 11, 2004

Today is my birthday. When I got up this morning, I thanked GOD for blessing me to see another year. I thanked him for being with me through these crises, but I'm in no mood to celebrate anything.

****

October 12, 2004

It's been five days already since Mama has eaten or drunk anything. I wonder how long she can go on like this.

The VITAS social worker and the clergyman came out this morning to talk to me and Daddy. The VITAS staff have been a godsend during Mama's sickness.

This afternoon, the nurse (Elizabeth Davis) came out; she could see that Daddy was having a hard time dealing with Mama's condition. Liz said maybe it would not be wise for Mama to stay at home until she died like we'd planned, because Daddy wasn't able to handle her suffering very well.

She suggested that we have Mama sent to Comfort Care at Miami Heart Hospital. The way Mama looked and sounded that day, I knew that it's getting close to the end for her.

I talked it over with Daddy and he agreed to have Mama admitted to the hospital, in the Comfort Care unit.

When the ambulance came, I rode to the hospital with Mama, but when the ambulance driver backed out of our driveway, I cried because I knew that Mama would never come home again.

Clara drove Daddy to the hospital later that night.

They stayed until Daddy start falling asleep. Clara took him home so that he'd be able to take his morning medication. I was packed and ready to stay for the long haul.

The next morning, Anon (Bobbie's son) came in and sat with me. Mama was still holding on.

By two o'clock, Saudia (Bobbie's daughter), her husband, and her three sons had come from Atlanta.

I was glad to see her boys. I had not seen Saudia's baby since she'd had him. I wished that it had been under different circumstances.

**************** *************

October 14, 2004

It's been two days now and Mama is still holding on. Daddy has been coming to the hospital every night, and so have Clara and Karen. I think that Mama's still hanging on because she hears our voices. Even until the end, she's being Mama — always there for her kids.

Mama's still not eating or drinking. She is just staring into space, but she could still hear us talking and crying for her.

A mother's instinct is to be there for her children, and although Mama is dying, she's still doing what comes naturally to her: she's holding on as long as she could hear her children crying for her.

But Mama was tired, and she needed rest. When we all went out to the lounge, I told everyone what I thought. I asked them to leave and not to return to the hospital room that evening.

I stayed the rest of the night. As I sat in the room with Mama, I told her to rest and that I'd make sure that Daddy would be okay, and that I'd be all right too. I told Mama that she could let go of this world and rest, because GOD was waiting for her.

*********************** ********************

October 15, 2004

I went to the desk down the hall from Mama's hospital room this morning and thanked everyone for keeping Mama comfortable and for comforting our family during our time of grief.

I told them that I was going to stay with Mama until noon, and I was going home. I went back into the room and packed up my things. I kissed Mama's face.

At twelve thirty, I went home.

At two thirty, the hospital called.

Mama was gone.

Although I knew that Mama was going to die and leave me, I still ached inside when I got the news. I was sad, but it was a relief that Mama was not suffering anymore. When I got off of the phone, I went in to tell Daddy. When I sat down next to him, he already knew what I was going to say; he just needed to hear the words.

"Daddy..." I said very softly, "that was the hospital calling. They said that Mama's just passed away."

At first, there was silence. Then Daddy let out a painful groaning sound. He got up and began to walk around the house and cried. I called Clara and told her that Mama was gone. Clara said that she would call Karen. I went into my room and closed the door and cried too.

My worst nightmare had been having Mama die and leave me in this world to live without her. Even as an adult, I had that fear, but Alzheimer's had taken Mama away from me even before she actually died. Losing a loved one to Alzheimer's is as devastating as losing them in death — or worse.

I thought about the prayer I had prayed as a kid when my friend's mother had died. The devastation she endured from her mother's death made me think of how devastated I'd be if anything ever happened to Mama.

As Mama went through the different stages of Alzheimer's, I suffered right along with her. It was very painful for me to watch Mama do and say things that I knew she would never have done had she known what she was doing. Alzheimer's was diminishing her mind and undoing everything she'd ever learned.

Daddy had been in denial and I couldn't talk to him about Mama's condition. Clara and Karen couldn't do anything about Mama's situation, to there was no use in getting them upset by telling them about everything Mama did, so I wrote in my journal and I prayed a lot.

I soon realized that GOD was all I needed when he was all I had to talk to.

There was a time when I didn't think I'd survive. But Mama did die, and it didn't kill me. Instead, I found strength and a peace I never encountered before. And yes, Mama did leave me, and I survived it. And as much as my heart ached, my endurance increased, and I thank GOD for strengthening me so that I could take care of Mama even until the end. In the days ahead, I know that I'll have painful reminders. My heart will break and my soul will ache, but I'll have a comfort that will see me through.

Days and even weeks had passed since Mama had died. Daddy was still crying and grieving over Mama's death. He was at Mama's gravesite almost all the time. I understood Daddy's grief: he had a lifetime partner for sixty-five years and now he had to adjust his life to her absence.

It must be devastating.

I collected all the pictures of Mama in the house and put them away for a while, at least until Mama's absence was more of a reality to Daddy. I know that he'll never get used to the fact that Mama is gone, but I'll just try to comfort him as best I can.

Friends and family still come by to say that they are sorry for our loss, or that they're sorry that we lost our mom. I thank them for their concern, but I don't see it as a loss: I know that on the day she took her last breath in this life, she began a new life in heaven.

THE END

****
****

In an effort to give Mama the very best care I knew how to give, I relied on GOD first, and when I needed comforting, I read Proverbs 3:5-6:

> Trust in the Lord
> with all thine
> heart; and lean
> not in thine own
> understanding.

In all thy ways, acknowledge him, and he shall direct thy paths.

Matthew 11:28:

Come unto me all ye that labour and are heavy laden, and I will give you rest.

These scriptures lift me up and gave me contentment.
****

I also searched and found a very reliable source of information in a book written by Davis Shenk, a national bestseller called The Forgetting (Alzheimer's: Portrait of an Epidemic).

I would encourage the loved ones and caregivers of Alzheimer's sufferers to buy David Shenk's book. It helped me to validate and confirm the stages of the Alzheimer's disease while I was taking care of Mama. Knowing more about what your loved ones are enduring helps reduce the heartbreaking and emotional stress we go through with them. When you read this book, you will know what to expect in all stages of the disease.

Alzheimer's disease shows no favor to anyone. It will invade the mind and memory of any race, social background, gender, or class. This disease is the worst thing that can happen to any human being who can think.
********************   ****************